Obstetrics

C000069542

Obstetrics

GEOFFREY CHAMBERLAIN

MD, FRCS, FRCOG, FACOG (Hon)
Professor of Obstetrics & Gynaecology
St George's Hospital Medical School
London

Seventh edition

Blackwell
Science

© 1962, 1966, 1975, 1980, 1984, 1992, 1996 by
Blackwell Science Ltd
Editorial Offices:
Osney Mead, Oxford OX2 0EL
25 John Street, London WCIN 2BL
23 Ainslie Place, Edinburgh EH3 6AJ
238 Main Street, Cambridge
    Massachusetts 02142, USA
54 University Street, Carlton
    Victoria 3053, Australia

Other Editorial Offices:
Arnette Blackwell SA
    224, Boulevard Saint Germain
    75007 Paris, France

Blackwell Wissenschafts-Verlag GmbH
    Kurfürstendamm 57
    10707 Berlin, Germany

    Zehetnergasse 6
    A-1140 Wien
    Austria

All rights reserved. No part of
this publication may be reproduced,
stored in a retrieval system, or
transmitted, in any form or by any
means, electronic, mechanical,
photocopying, recording or otherwise,
except as permitted by the UK
Copyright, Designs and Patents Act
1988, without the prior permission
of the copyright owner.

First published 1962
Reprinted 1964
Second edition 1966
Reprinted 1968
Third edition 1975
Reprinted 1976
Fourth edition 1980
Portuguese translation 1980
Reprinted 1981, 1983
Fifth edition 1984
Italian translation 1984
Sixth edition 1992
Reprinted 1993
Four Dragons edition 1992
Reprinted 1993
Seventh edition 1996
International edition 1996

Set by Excel Typesetters Co., Hong Kong
Printed and bound in Great Britain
at the University Press, Cambridge

The Blackwell Science logo is a
trade mark of Blackwell Science Ltd,
registered at the United Kingdom
Trade Marks Registry

DISTRIBUTORS

Marston Book Services Ltd
PO Box 269
Abingdon
Oxon OX14 4YN
(Orders: Tel: 01235 465500
        Fax: 01235 465555)

USA
Blackwell Science, Inc.
238 Main Street
Cambridge, MA 02142
(Orders: Tel: 800 215-1000
        617 876-7000
        Fax: 617 492-5263)

Canada
Copp Clark, Ltd
2775 Matheson Blvd East
Mississauga, Ontario
Canada, L4W 4P7
(Orders: Tel: 800 263-4374
        905 238-6074)

Australia
Blackwell Science Pty Ltd
54 University Street
Carlton, Victoria 3053
(Orders: Tel: 03 9347 0300
        Fax: 03 9349 3016)

A catalogue record for this title
is available from the British Library

ISBN 0-86542-681-3 (BSL)
     0-86542-699-6 (International Edition)

Library of Congress
Cataloging-in-publication Data

Chamberlain, Geoffrey, 1930.
    Lecture notes on obstetrics /
    Geoffrey Chamberlain.—7th ed.
        p.   cm.
    Includes bibliographical references
and index.
    Cover title: Obstetrics.
    ISBN 0-86542-681-3
    1. Obstetrics—Handbooks, manuals, etc.
I. Title. II. Title: Obstetrics
    [DNLM: 1. Obstetrics.   WQ 100 C443L
1996]
RG 531.C45   1996
618.2—dc20
DNLM/DLC
for Library of Congress   96-11891
                                CIP

Contents

Preface to the Seventh Edition

The science of obstetrics increases rapidly. This has led to a revision of the last edition which was prepared in 1990. New technologies are improving our ability to detect problems; we now need to work on the treatment of these problems and their prevention. This is the phase of medicine that follows diagnosis, but we cannot proceed with therapy without diagnosis first. In all this, the art of the subject still goes on. More thought is now given to the woman and her place in pregnancy and childbirth. The midwife's role has been enhanced in the last few years, quite rightly. All this is reflected in this seventh edition. I have retained much of the physiological background throughout the book, which is needed to understand the changes. We have reduced the length by removing the section on contraception which can be found in *Lecture Notes on Gynaecology* and by dealing only with those parts of neonatal paediatrics which concern the obstetrician. A very good account of the diagnosis and care of the abnormal newborn is in *Lecture Notes on Neonatology*.

I have written this book primarily for medical students sitting MB BS, but it is sufficiently comprehensive and would be useful for the DRCOG examination. Midwives in the past have found these lecture notes helpful and I have borne this in mind in the preparation of this seventh edition. I am grateful to Mrs Sue Cunningham, my Personal Assistant at St George's Hospital for many years. She has most patiently dealt with the various material that I have prepared. I am also grateful to my publishers at Blackwell Science for their work and particularly to Andrew Robinson, the Commissioning Editor, and Alice Emmott, the Production Editor, both of whom have been of much assistance throughout.

Geoffrey Chamberlain
Swansea 1996

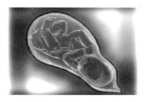

Normal Anatomy and Physiology

Reproduction

Life begins when an oocyte is fertilized by a sperm.

The oocyte is expelled from the ovary about mid-cycle when the fimbriated end of the Fallopian tube, possibly excited by chemotaxis, closes to embrace the ovary like a hand holding a rugby football. The egg has virtually no transperitoneal passage.

At the time of intercourse millions of sperms are deposited in the vagina. They travel in all directions, some through the cervix where, in midcycle, the molecules of cervical mucus untangle their barbed-wire-like morphology to assume straight lines. A few sperm reach each Fallopian tube where they swim counter-current, the first arriving near the oocyte within 30 minutes of intercourse. One sperm only penetrates the zona pellucida by hyaluronidase activity; the tail is shed, the sperm's neck becomes the centrosome and the head is the male pronucleus containing half the genetic potential of the future fetus.

Fertilization usually occurs at the ampullary end of the Fallopian tube within 12–24 hours of the oocyte production. The fertilized egg then travels along the tube propelled by:
- Muscular peristalsis of the tube.
- Currents in tube fluid whipped by cilia.

During this time, nutrition and oxygenation is from the fluid secreted by the glandular cells of the Fallopian tube lining. Arriving in the uterus 4–5 days later, it is in the cavity for 2–3 days and implants in the thick endometrium in the secretory phase on about day 22 of the cycle. The blastocyst starts to put out pseudopodia so that the surface area available for maternofetal exchange is increased. All transfer is by osmosis and diffusion at this stage.

Early fetal development

Fetal development is well documented in most mammalian species including the human.

Since many women cannot time the precise act of coitus at which fertilization occurred, it is conventional to date pregnancy in weeks from the 1st day of the last normal menstrual period (LNMP). The difference in the clinical timing of pregnancy and biological age (from conception) is readily understood on realizing that no-one becomes pregnant in the first half of a menstrual cycle. The first 14 days of pregnancy do not exist using the 1st day of the last normal menstrual period as a method of timing (Fig. 1.1).

The following milestones are particularly important.

Four weeks (from LNMP) or 14 days biological life
- Sac 2–3 mm.
- Ectoderm ⎫
- Mesoderm ⎬ formed.
- Endoderm ⎭
- Yolk sac formed.

Six weeks (from LNMP)
- Sac 20–25 mm; embryo 10 mm—can be seen on ultrasound.
- A cylinder with head and tail end formed.
- Pulsation of heart tube.
- Body stalk (umbilical cord) formed.
- Villi appear in cytotrophoblast.

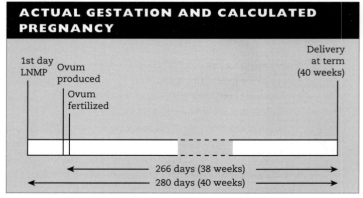

Fig. 1.1 The differences between the actual length of gestation and the calculated length of pregnancy from the LNMP.

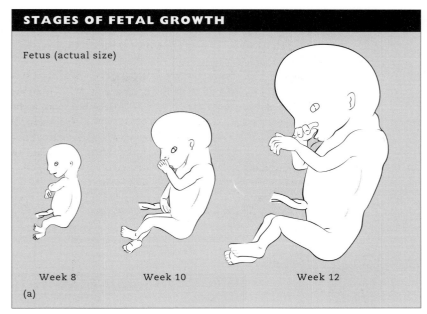

STAGES OF FETAL GROWTH

Fetus (actual size)

Week 8   Week 10   Week 12

(a)

Fig. 1.2 Different stages of fetal growth. (a) Actual size of the fetus at 8, 10 and 12 weeks. (*Continued on p. 4.*)

Eight weeks (from LNMP)
- Sac 30–50 mm; fetus 25 mm (Fig. 1.2).
- Sex glands differentiated.
- Limbs well formed, toes and fingers present.
- Centres of ossification present.

Twelve weeks (from LNMP)
- Sac 100 mm; fetus 90 mm.
- Primary development of all organ systems.
- Nails on fingers and toes.

Early placental development

The placenta (Fig. 1.3) is formed from:
- Chorion   ⎤
- Decidua basalis ⎦ covered by amnion.

Villi are buds from chorionic plate. At first they are made of cytotro-

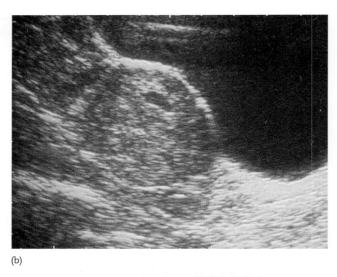

(b)

Fig. 1.2 (*Cont.*)
Different stages of
fetal growth. (b)
Ultrasound showing a
sac at 6 weeks. (c)
Ultrasound showing a
sac and fetus at 8
weeks (between +
and +).

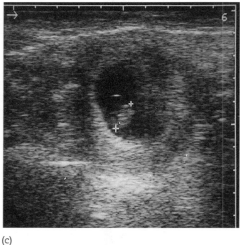

(c)

phoblast tissue only. Mesoderm appears *in situ* in the centre of the core of
each villus (Fig. 1.4).

In this mesodermal core, angioblastic strands are formed. The cells on
the edge of these become the endothelium of blood vessels and the central cells, the red blood cells. The vessels of the villus join the vessels

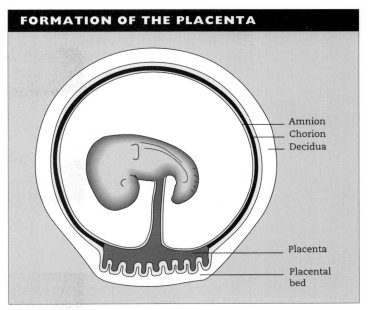

Fig. 1.3 Formation of placenta in relation to fetus and fetal membranes.

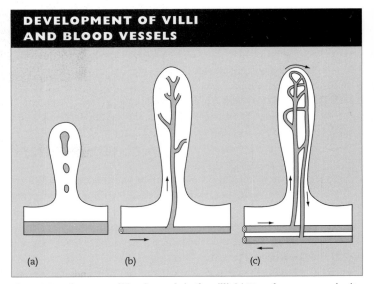

Fig. 1.4 Development of blood vessels in the villi. (a) Mesoderm appears *in situ* in the core of a villus of proliferating trophoblast cells. (b) Blood vessels form and join up with those in the mesoderm layer. (c) Capillaries from arterial side circulate blood back to veins.

formed in the mesoderm. By 22 days, the fetal heart pumps blood and a functioning circulation starts.

By 8 weeks, the villi are 200 µm in diameter with a well-organized circulatory system and a double layer of epithelium (cytotrophoblast or Langhans' layer covered by a cellular syncytiotrophoblast).

Further demands of fetal metabolism require swifter exchange at the placenta. These come as a result of:

1 Longer and larger villi ⎫ therefore greater surface area.
2 Branching of villi   ⎭

3 Absorption of Langhans' layer so that syncytiotrophoblast is in direct contact with blood capillary.

4 Syncytiotrophoblast thinned and nuclei migrate from areas over capillaries where exchange actually occurs.

5 Localized dome-like swellings occur on the villi protruding into the intervillous space. These areas are especially thin-walled and are probably the site of much of the gas exchange.

Villi are like fronds of seaweed under water as the maternal blood circulates around them (Fig. 1.5). As the placenta grows, fetal size is proportional to the surface area available for exchange at first. The number of stem villi do not increase after the 12th week. Hence the number of lobules is now fixed. The rest of growth is by proliferation and by growth of old peripheral villi.

Fetal physiology

The major functions will be reviewed particularly where they differ from adult physiological patterns.

CARDIOVASCULAR SYSTEM

The heart is beating by 22 days and can be detected with vaginal ultrasound at 5 weeks (from LNMP).

There are bypasses in the system since the lungs are not used; less than 10% of blood goes through them (Fig. 1.6).

Umbilical blood flow increases with fetal weight. This increase is disproportionate but with enhanced O_2 carrying capacity of the fetal blood, the total O_2 transport is increased. Flow is about 100 ml/kg/min, as measured experimentally, but may be greater in the body *in vivo*.

Fetal haemoglobin

HbA (adult haemoglobin) differs from HbF (fetal haemoglobin) by a 25% alteration of amino acid radicals in chains. At any given PO_2, the O_2 dissociation curve of HbF is to the left of HbA so it has greater O_2 affinity (Fig.

CIRCULATION OF MATERNAL BLOOD

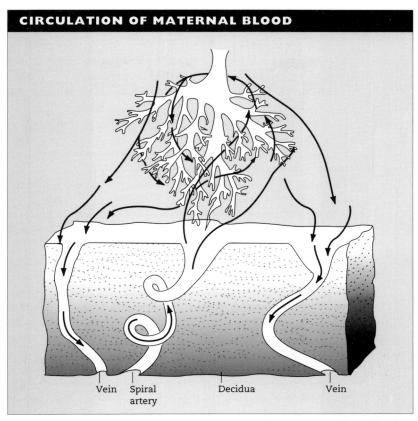

Fig. 1.5 Circulation of maternal blood around fine exchange villi and showing one anchoring villus.

1.7). The fetus has higher Hb concentration than the adult (18 g/dl of blood compared with 13 g/dl) allowing further O_2 uptake at placenta and greater release to tissues. Production of HbF diminishes before birth and has usually stopped by a year later (Fig. 1.8).

RESPIRATORY SYSTEM

This has to adjust within 1–2 minutes from an intrauterine to an independent state. Vascular loops occur in the lungs by 18 weeks. Alveoli develop by 22 weeks.

Surface tension of alveolar epithelium is decreased by surfactant lipoproteins, which are not present in immature fetuses. Hence if they are

FETAL AND NEONATAL CIRCULATION

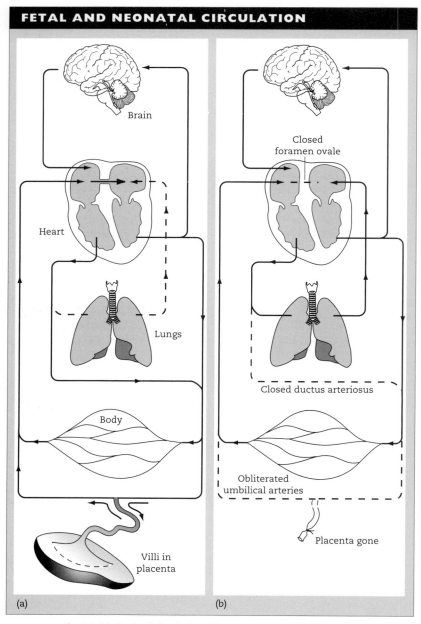

Fig. 1.6 (a) The fetal circulation. (b) The neonatal circulation. Note closure of bypasses after birth.

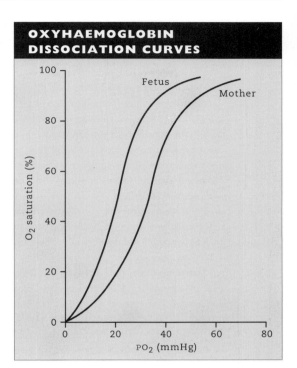

Fig. 1.7 Oxyhaemoglobin dissociation curves for human maternal and fetal blood at pH 7.4 and 37°C.

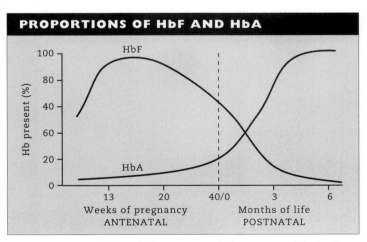

Fig. 1.8 Proportion of HbF and HbA present at different stages of fetal and postnatal life.

born prematurely it is difficult to open up their lungs and the respiratory distress syndrome occurs.

Production of surfactant increases after 34 weeks. This is particularly true of sphingomyelin, more than lecithin, and so the ratio between them alters sharply between 32 and 36 weeks (Fig. 1.9).

Before birth, the alveoli are closed and the trachea is filled with lung fluid which is different from amniotic fluid and is secreted from glandular cells in the periphery of the bronchiolar system. Small spontaneous respiratory movements occur, but if the fetus is made hypoxic, larger efforts are made; then (and only then) amniotic fluid is drawn into the trachea. Most non-stressed infants are born with a respiratory tract filled with lung fluid, not amniotic fluid.

Fetal development is mostly by growth (Fig. 1.10); most congenital defects that are going to occur will have been formed by 10 weeks. The critical periods in the development of the human embryo are shown in Fig. 1.11.

Growing from one cell to six billion demands organization of cells into functioning systems so that all can metabolize under optimal conditions. The rate of growth is greatest in the first weeks. Cellular increase is under the control of maternal and fetal hormones; at first, oestrogens are most influential, then later insulin-like growth factors. In very early pregnancy oestrogens regulate the supply of nutrients in

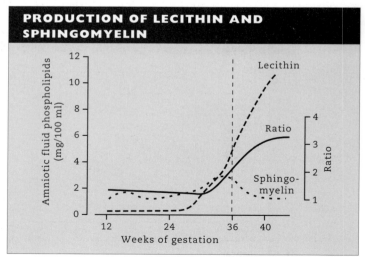

Fig. 1.9 Production of lecithin and sphingomyelin through pregnancy and the ratio between these substances.

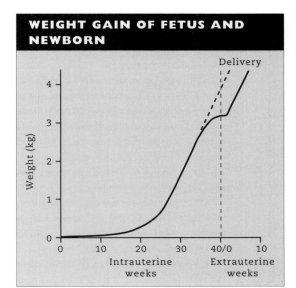

Fig. 1.10 The weight gain of the fetus and newborn child. The growth potential falls off in the last few weeks of pregnancy. Note that, after the immediate weight drop, neonatal growth continues at the same incremental rate as it did in the uterus.

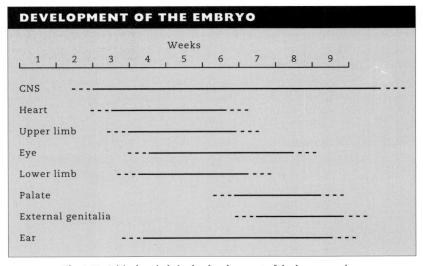

Fig. 1.11 Critical periods in the development of the human embryo. Abnormalities are likely to follow if appropriate teratogens act on tissues at these sensitive times.

uterine fluid. Later they regulate the course of the blood supply to the placental bed.

After mid-pregnancy, growth is also determined by placental transfer. This could be impaired by:

1 A low environment supply from the mother of:
  • Oxygen—only has effect in last weeks, e.g. living at high altitudes.
  • Nutrients—only shows with extremes of starvation.

2 Reduced blood flow to the placental bed. This follows lack of normal invasion of the arcuate arteries by trophoblasts at 22 weeks. This is estimated by Doppler ultrasound.

3 Poor exchange across the syncytiotrophoblast membrane; if this should be reduced a smaller baby results.

Ultimately growth is determined by:

1 Genetic factors inherited from both parents.

2 Placental transfer of nutrients dependent on:
  • Placental bed flow rates.
  • Placental membrane transfer.

Placental physiology

Exchange

The placenta is the fetal exchange station. Compare Fig. 1.12a and Fig. 1.12b. Figure 1.12a is an adult with organs of homeostasis (kidney, skin and lung) communicating with the outside environment—the air in the case of humans. Figure 1.12b shows the fetal situation where these same homeostatic organs only communicate with the amniotic sac—a closed cavity. All exchange must take place via the placenta to the mother and thence (using her kidneys, skin and lungs) to the outside. The placenta is called the lung of the fetus but is also its liver and kidneys.

Placental hormones

The placenta has a second set of functions, that of an endocrine organ making hormones that regulate the following:

1 Rate of growth of fetus:
  • At first directly.
  • Later indirectly through control of placental bed blood supply.

2 Activity of uterus to:
  • Prevent premature expulsion of fetus.
  • Encourage labour contractions at correct time.

3 Activity of other organs:
  • Breasts.

FETAL ENVIRONMENT

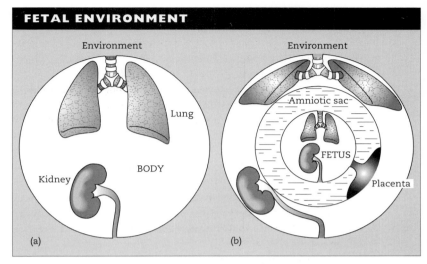

Fig. 1.12 (a) Non-pregnant woman. (b) The fetal environment in the pregnant woman.

- Ligaments of pelvis in pregnancy.

The hormones made by the placenta are detailed below.

Chorionic gonadotrophin

Made in: Langhans' cells.

Function: prolong corpus luteum (early);

may control progesterone metabolism (late).

Oestrogens

Made in: all tissues of placenta.

Function: stimulate uterine growth and development.

Progesterone

Made in: cytotrophoblast.

Function: damp down intrinsic uterine action in pregnancy and protect placental bed;

may guard fetus from high cortisol effects (potassium-retaining).

Human placental lactogen

Made in: syncytiotrophoblast.

Function: alters glucose and insulin metabolism;
               may initiate lactation.

Placental tissues age. Maximum efficiency is at 37–38 weeks; many functions deteriorate after this.

Beware extrapolations between these two groups of functions of the placenta—transfer and endocrine. The correlations may not be valid.

The fetus and placenta at term

THE FETUS

The anatomical features of the fetus which most concern the obstetrician are those found in the mature fetus after 36 weeks' gestation. The most important area is that which is largest, hardest and most difficult to deliver —the head.

The head

Certain measurements should be remembered (Fig. 1.13). These diameters engage in the maternal pelvic brim at different degrees of flexion of the fetal head on the neck.

The intracranial arrangement of meninges is important (Fig. 1.14) for, under stress, it can be damaged to produce intracranial haemorrhage.

The body

The rest of the fetus will usually pass where the head leads. The bisacromial diameter of the shoulders is about 10 cm.

PLACENTA

A discoid with lobules (15–20) packed together.

Fetal surface

Covered with amnion (not chorion which fuses with edge). Fetal vessels (arteries paler than veins) course over it diving into each lobule as an end vessel.

Maternal surface

Lobules of compressed villi (like seaweed out of water) separated from each other by sulci.

Types of cord insertion (Fig. 1.15)

For types of cord insertion see Fig. 1.15.

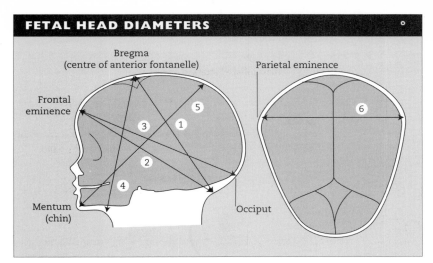

Fig. 1.13 The important diameters of the fetal head of a 3-kg baby:

1 Suboccipitobregmatic 10 cm ⎫ Present with various degrees
2 Suboccipitofrontal 11 ⎬ of flexion of a cephalic
3 Occipitofrontal 12 ⎭ presentation.
4 Submentobregmatic 10 ⎫ Present with brow presentation
5 Mentovertical 13 ⎬ Present with extension of a
6 Biparietal 10. ⎭ face presentation.

CEREBRAL VEINS IN THE MENINGES

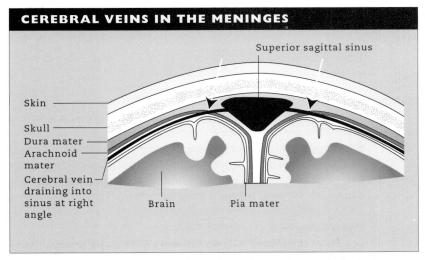

Fig. 1.14 Arrangement of the meninges showing how cerebral veins traverse them. If much intracranial movement occurs, the arachnoid moves with the brain but the dura stays with the skull. Hence the vein can be torn at the arrowed sites.

TYPES OF CORD INSERTION

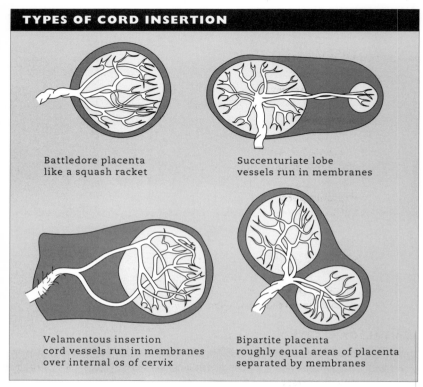

Battledore placenta
like a squash racket

Succenturiate lobe
vessels run in membranes

Velamentous insertion
cord vessels run in membranes
over internal os of cervix

Bipartite placenta
roughly equal areas of placenta
separated by membranes

Fig. 1.15 Types of cord insertion.

Maternal side of the placental circulation

Maternal blood is in vessels in the placental bed. It is temporarily in contact with foreign tissues (syncytiotrophoblast of villi) outside the endothelium. Spiral arteries (about 200) lead blood from the uterine arteries to
the placental bed pool. Maternal blood spurts under arterial blood pressure, loses way against a mass of villi and passes laterally, pushed by *vis a
tergo* to the placental bed veins scattered over the floor of the placental
bed and not grouped into marginal sinuses in the human. Such flow patterns can be shown by cine-angioradiography.

Measurement of blood flow to the placental bed has been very difficult
because it involved direct measurement in animals (unphysiological) or
indirect methods with electromagnetic flow meters in man (imprecise).
Now indirect measurements with Doppler ultrasound allow more precise
non-invasive flow studies in man.

Maternal blood flow to uterus is 100–150 ml/kg/min in late pregnancy, of which 80–85% goes to the placenta.

Abnormal implantation

Placenta accreta
Villi penetrate decidua just into the myometrial layer; difficulty in separation.

Placenta increta
Villi penetrate deeply into myometrium. Even more difficult to separate.

Placenta percreta
Villi penetrate to subperitoneal myometrium. Impossible to separate.

The three diagnoses above cannot be differentiated clinically. They are pathological ones made at sectioning a uterus after removal.

Placenta praevia
Implantation in the lower segment of the uterus.

UMBILICAL CORD
At term about 50-cm long, 2-cm in diameter. Contains two arteries and a vein which is derived from the left umbilical vein of the embryo. (The right one usually disappears.)

Arteries spiral and give a cordlike appearance. Possibly their pattern wrapped around the vein allows their pulsations to help massage blood back along the umbilical vein. The vessels are packed and protected by a viscous fluid—Wharton's jelly.

There are no nerves in the cord or placenta. Hence ligation and cutting the umbilical cord does not hurt the fetus.

AMNIOTIC FLUID
This surrounds the fetus.

Produced:	in early pregnancy: from amnion over placenta and sac;
	in late pregnancy: from fetal urine as well.
Volume:	increase to 38 weeks;
	500–1500 ml.
Osmolality:	decreases in late pregnancy.
Creatinine:	increases in late pregnancy.

DIAGNOSTIC USES OF CHECKING AMNIOTIC FLUID

1 α-Fetoprotein levels for open central nervous system (CNS) abnormalities.
2 Chromosome content of amniocytes and fetal skin cells in genetic diseases.
3 Rhesus effect measuring bilirubin breakdown products.
4 Metabolic upset of the fetus.
5 Infection of the amniotic cavity in premature rupture of membranes.
6 Respiratory maturity by measuring the lecithin–sphingomyelin ratio.

Box 1.1 Diagnostic uses of checking amniotic fluid.

Acid–base: normally accumulation of CO_2 and fixed acid causes a slight reduction in pH (about 7.15–7.20).

Amniotic fluid can be removed at amniocentesis and used diagnostically to check a number of factors (Box 1.1).

Maternal anatomy in pregnancy

UTERUS

A hollow, muscle-walled organ in the pelvis communicating with each Fallopian tube and, through its cervix, the vagina.

Pre-pregnancy: $7 \times 5 \times 3$ cm—40 g.
Full term: $30 \times 25 \times 20$ cm—1000 g.

Structure (Fig. 1.16)

Muscle in three layers with vascular anastomosis between.

1 Outer: thin, longitudinal, merging with ligaments.
2 Middle: very thick, spiral muscle fibres with blood vessels between.
3 Inner: thin, oblique with condensation at each cornu and at the upper and lower end of the cervical canal (sphincters).

Increase in size during pregnancy mostly due to hypertrophy of existing cells rather than increase in number. Changes stimulated by oestrogen and gradual stretch (maximum effective stretch about term).

Blood supply

From the uterine and ovarian arteries, mostly the former. These hypertrophy so that, by term, a litre of blood can be in the uterine vasculature. Branches increase in size, number and diameter from each side of uterus (little mid-line crossing). Placental site gets preferential blood supply. Penetrating branches pass through myometrium; under the surface of the

RELATIONS OF THE UTERUS

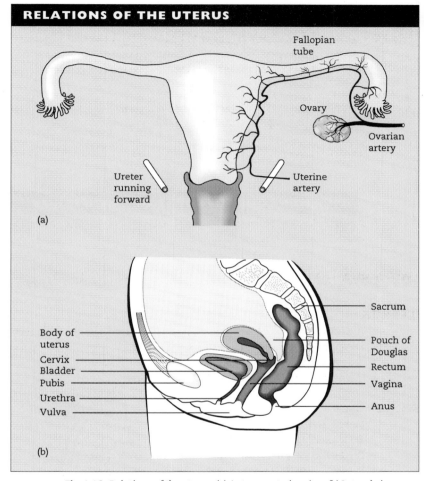

Fig. 1.16   Relations of the uterus. (a) Anteroposterior view. (b) Lateral view.

decidua they become spiral arteries and then penetrate the decidua. In early pregnancy their exits into the placental bed pool are narrow but tro-phoblast invasion after 16 weeks normally widens them into deltas so reducing resistance and improving flow. If invasion is incomplete, flow is restricted so that:

- In late pregnancy, the fetus gets less nutrients for growth.
- In labour, the fetus gets less O_2 and so fetal distress follows more readily.

Cervix

Barrel-shaped canal at the bottom of the uterus. Mostly connective tissue with muscle at upper and lower end (internal and external sphincters). As ground substance of connective tissue becomes softer with a greater water content under the influences of oestrogens, the cervix becomes softer clinically.

Ligaments

Uterus supported by ligaments (Fig. 1.17). In pregnancy these are stretched and thickened. They soften because of the progesterone and relaxin effect on collagen.

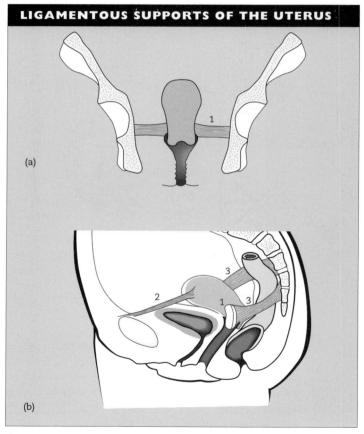

LIGAMENTOUS SUPPORTS OF THE UTERUS

(a)

(b)

Fig. 1.17 The ligamentous supports of the uterus. (a) Frontal view. (b) Lateral view. 1, Cardinal ligaments; 2, round ligaments; 3, uterosacral ligaments.

BONY PELVIS

False pelvis is to true pelvis like a saucer on top of a cup. The true pelvis is important obstetrically, the false pelvis is not. Diameters are shown in Fig. 1.18.

The longest axis of the pelvis changes through 90° going from top to bottom. Hence anything passing through must rotate.

Long curved posterior wall, short anterior wall. Hence anything passing through takes a curved course (Fig. 1.19).

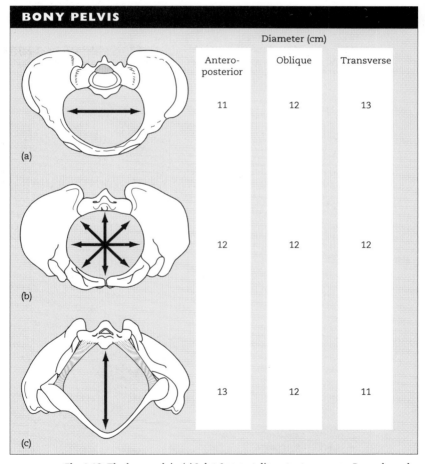

BONY PELVIS

	Diameter (cm)		
	Antero-posterior	Oblique	Transverse
(a)	11	12	13
(b)	12	12	12
(c)	13	12	11

Fig. 1.18 The bony pelvis. (a) Inlet. Longest diameter transverse. Bean shaped. (b) Mid-cavity. All diameters equal. Circle. (c) Outlet. Longest diameter antero-posterior. Diamond shaped.

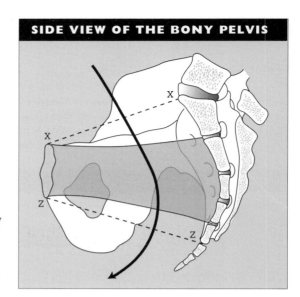

SIDE VIEW OF THE BONY PELVIS

Fig. 1.19 Side view of bony pelvis, showing the plane of the inlet (x–x), the zone of the mid-cavity (toned), and the plane of the outlet (z–z).

The three bones — two ilia and a sacrum — are held together at joints by ligaments which soften in pregnancy allowing play at these sites.

The coccyx is a fused group of the last vertebrae, hinged on sacrum by a joint which easily allows bending back in childbirth.

PELVIC MUSCLES

Consider in three groups.

Lining lateral wall of pelvis
- Pyriformis.
- Obturator internus.

Make pelvic diaphragm
- Levator ani.
- Coccygeus.

Beneath pelvic diaphragm
I   Anterior triangle.
   - Deep perineal: compressor urethrae; deep transverse perinei.
   - Superficial perineal: ischiocavernosus; bulbocavernosus; superficial transverse perinei.

2 Posterior triangle.
  • Sphincter ani.

Essentials of pelvic musculature

1 The pyriformis muscles reduce the useful transverse diameter of upper and mid-cavities, thus thrusting the fetus forward.

2 The pelvic diaphragm and its fascia are like a pair of cupped hands tilted slightly forward (Fig. 1.20). Muscle fibres lace from the one hand to the other, being especially thick around the three tubes which broach and so weaken the diaphragm, the urethra, the vagina and the rectum. These slings of muscle can pull each of the tubes forward to make a voluntary extra sphincter mechanism.

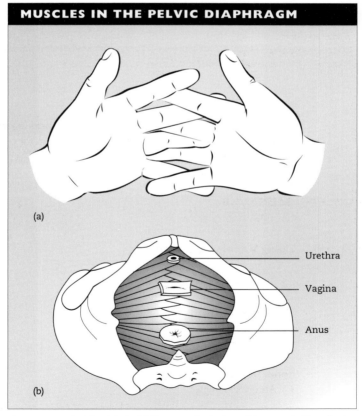

MUSCLES IN THE PELVIC DIAPHRAGM

(a)

Urethra

Vagina

Anus

(b)

Fig. 1.20 Interlocking hands (a) illustrate the lacing of the muscle fibres in the pelvic diaphragm (b).

3 With an episiotomy or a moderate obstetric tear, the pelvic diaphragm is rarely involved. The perineal body and the perineal muscles inserted into it usually are damaged or cut but not higher structures.

BREASTS

Each has 15–20 separate racemose glands leading via a duct to the nipple (Fig. 1.21).

Changes in pregnancy

The glands enlarge because:
- Increase in gland substance under influence of progesterone.
- Increase in fat between gland masses under influence of oestrogens.
- Skin of areola darkened under influence of melanocyte-stimulating hormone released by pituitary.
- Nipples become softer because of progesterone effect on connective tissue.
- Sebaceous glands increase (Montgomery tubercles) possibly as a result of oestrogen secretion.

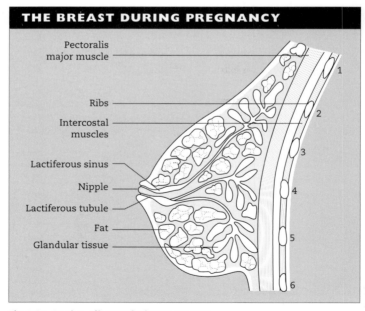

THE BREAST DURING PREGNANCY

Pectoralis major muscle — 1
Ribs — 2
Intercostal muscles — 3
Lactiferous sinus —
Nipple — 4
Lactiferous tubule —
Fat — 5
Glandular tissue — 6

Fig. 1.21 Section of breast during pregnancy.

Maternal physiology in pregnancy

Pregnancy causes alterations not just in the mother's pelvis and abdomen but affects the whole body. Adaptations in the function of various systems occur to minimize the stresses imposed; these are interlinked smoothly and the function of the whole organism does not deteriorate—when any natural system in dynamic equilibrium is put under constraint, the system moves in such a way as to remove that constraint. In a healthy pregnancy, the constraint is *not* the fetus alone but the effects on maternal physiology caused by the fetus and placenta.

METABOLISM

Increased to provide for:

- Increased growth of fetus and placenta.
- Increased growth of containing organs.
- Increased growth of support systems.
- Preparation for lactation.

Weight increase (Table 1.1)

Usually 10–14 kg (22–30 lb) in whole pregnancy. For example:

0–14 weeks: 2 kg (4.5 lb)—may be a loss because of vomiting;

13–28 weeks: 5 kg (11 lb);

28–40 weeks: 5 kg (11 lb)—may be a loss in last 2–3 weeks because of diminution of amniotic fluid.

The rest is extracellular fluid, fat and protein stroage—6 kg, (very variable average).

A sharp increase in the mother's weight gain in late pregnancy may indicate increased water retention, a facet of pre-eclampsia. Weight loss, if persistent, may reflect poor fetal progress and may indicate more

Table 1.1 Breakdown of approximate weight increase during pregnancy.

WEIGHT INCREASE DURING PREGNANCY		
Fetus	3.5 kg	7 lb
Placenta	0.5	1
Amniotic fluid	1.5	2
Uterus	1.0	2
Blood increase	1.5	3
Breasts	1.0	2
Total	9.0 kg	17 lb

thorough surveillance although there is little precision in this and many obstetricians do not use it as a measure of well-being.

Protein

Fetus requires little protein in first half of pregnancy therefore negative balance.

Two-thirds of protein acquired in last 12 weeks (a half in last 4 weeks). Also maternal uterus and breasts use much protein in growing tissues and storage occurs against lactation. Approximately 12 g of nitrogen a day are needed for the development of these and of the fetus.

Carbohydrate

Pregnancy is diabetogenic (i.e. an increased resistance to insulin). Requirements of calories slightly increased.

Fat

Fetus increases fat content late. From 2% of the fetal body weight at 32 weeks, the proportion of fat increases to 12% at term. This is preceded by a greater absorption of fat by the mother and a higher circulating maternal lipid and lipoprotein level.

Calcium

Fetus utilizes calcium late, withdrawing it from storage depots in the trabeculae of long bones of the mother. If the stores are insufficient the fetus still utilizes calcium so leading to maternal osteomalacia. Despite this, maternal serum calcium levels stay steady.

Iron

Iron is mostly passed to the fetus in the last weeks of pregnancy where it is stored in the liver and other haemopoietic organs. The mother may have low stores of iron by then because of:
- Too little in diet, therefore give supplements.
- Too poor absorption, therefore make sure enough is in gut to be absorbed when required.

CARDIOVASCULAR SYSTEM

Load

Pregnancy is an increased load therefore increased work is required by the heart.
- Growing fetal tissues which have high O_2 consumption rates.
- Hypertrophied uterus and breasts require more O_2.

• Increased muscular effort by mother to cope with weight gain of 10–14 kg (22–30 lb).
• In last weeks of pregnancy, the placental bed may act like an arteriovenous fistula. More work is required to overcome this shunt.

Cardiac output

Increased needs are met by increasing cardiac output.

Cardiac output = stroke volume × pulse rate.

In pregnancy, pulse rate is raised and further increase comes from larger stroke output because of enlarged heart chambers and cardiac muscle hypertrophy.

Output increases rapidly in the first trimester by up to 40%. It does not peak at 30–32 weeks as was previously considered when incorrect measurements were used to determine output (Fig. 1.22).

During labour, cardiac output can increase by a further 2 l/min in association with uterine contractions.

Systolic blood pressure is a little low in pregnancy but diastolic pressure is much lower in early and mid-pregnancy, rising in last trimester. Peripheral resistance is decreased and since cardiac output is raised pulse pressure is increased.

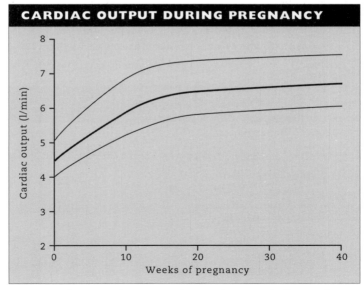

Fig. 1.22 Cardiac output in pregnancy in normal women. The lines on the graph represent the mean ±2 SD of the mean.

Blood volume

Return of blood to the heart is maintained by increased blood volume. Plasma volume increases more than red cell manufacture so that relative haemodilution occurs. This used to be called physiological anaemia but this is a bad term, for no pathological process can be physiological. This relative haemodilution may be one of the causes of increased fatigue in early and mid-pregnancy.

Heart changes

Pregnancy is a hyperkinetic state. The heart is:
- Enlarged.
- Pushed up.
- Unfolded upon aorta.

These changes produce electrocardiogram (ECG) and X-ray changes which are normal for pregnancy, but may appear pathological if interpreted without knowledge of pregnancy.

There are also sometimes extra murmurs, which are normal hypervolaemic sounds:
- Systolic ejection murmur.
- Third heart sound.
- Internal mammary artery murmur along the edge of sternum.

RESPIRATORY SYSTEM

Pressure of the growing uterus forces the diaphragm up and lower ribs out but vital capacity is not reduced in late pregnancy (Fig. 1.23).

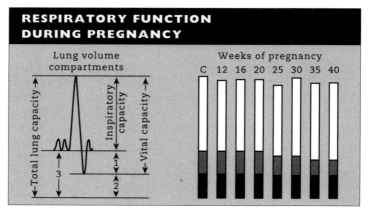

Fig. 1.23 The changes in respiratory function during pregnancy. 1, expiratory reserve volume; 2, residual volume; 3, functional residual volume.

Increased vascularity of mucous membrane makes greater mucus secretion in pregnancy and so there is often a flare up of ear, nose and throat problems.

URINARY TRACT

Renal function
- Renal plasma flow increases by 30–50%.
- Glomerular filtration rate increases by 30–50%.
- Tubular re-absorption increases by 30–50%.
- Patchy glomerular leak happens occasionally (e.g. glucose).

Lower urinary tract
- Bladder more irritated as growing uterus pushes on it.
- Ureters:
  - (a) Longer, wider, lower tone because of progesterone effects.
  - (b) Stasis in ureter and pelvis of kidney may lead to infection.

ALIMENTARY TRACT
- Hyperosmia
- Increased salivation } may lead to bizarre dietary habits (pica).
- Teeth more susceptible to spreading caries and gingivitis because of increased cortisone levels.
- Nausea and vomiting.
- Hypomotility of gut may lead to constipation.
- Hypochlorhydria because of regurgitation of alkaline chyle from intestine back into stomach.
- Slow emptying of gall bladder.

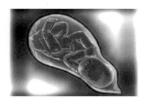

Antenatal Care and Intrauterine Welfare

The aims of antenatal care are to bring the mother and child to labour in the best possible condition. They are:

1 A screening process applied to the entire pregnant population to detect sub-groups at higher risk for complications of pregnancy.

2 Suitable diagnostic procedures to determine who are really at risk.

3 The management of high-risk pregnancies.

4 The educational preparation of the couple for childbirth and the rearing of the infant.

Diagnosis of pregnancy

SYMPTOMS

Amenorrhoea

The monthly shedding of the endometrium is prevented by the persistence of the corpus luteum which secretes progesterone. Pregnancy is dated from the 1st day of the LNMP even though conception does not occur until about 14 days later. Any bleeding after the LNMP should be considered as abnormal.

Nausea and vomiting

Approximately two-thirds of nulliparae and about one-half of multiparae experience nausea or vomiting to varying degrees. For many pregnant women this is the first sign of pregnancy with the symptoms occurring even before the first period is missed.

The vomiting usually completely disappears by 16 weeks' gestation and lessens in severity after about 12 weeks. Although some women are sick first thing in the morning, it is not unusual to find that vomiting may occur at any time of the day. Commonly some biscuits or sweets help prevent nausea.

There is usually no accompanying metabolic upset, women do not feel ill all the time, and it does not affect their daily activities.

Breast symptoms

Breast enlargement accompanied by tingling of the nipples may occur from the first missed period. Montgomery's tubercles develop from between 6 and 8 weeks' gestation and colostrum may be secreted from the nipples after about 12 weeks' gestation.

Urinary symptoms

From 6 weeks' gestation onwards, many women experience increased frequency of micturition. This is due to:
- Increased renal blood flow in the early stages.
- Pressure on the bladder from the growing uterus in later pregnancy.

SIGNS

Uterus

- An increased softness and a feeling that the uterus is cystic by 6–8 weeks' gestation.
- Increased size can be determined by bimanual vaginal examination from about 8 weeks onwards.

Breasts

- Increased in size and feel warm.
- The areolae darken.
- Montgomery's tubercles develop.
- Tortuous skin veins dilate.

INVESTIGATIONS

Pregnancy test

Animal pregnancy tests and early crude immunological tests have now been replaced by accurate, sensitive tests involving monoclonal antibodies.

Tests for β sub-unit hCG

Human chorionic gonadotrophin (hCG) is a glycoprotein hormone that contains two carbohydrate side chains: alpha (α) and beta (β). The α sub-unit is identical to that of follicle-stimulating hormone (FSH), luteinizing hormone (LH) and thyrotrophin (TSH). The β sub-unit is immunologically specific. hCG is secreted by the trophoblast cells of the fertilized ovum and later by the definitive placenta.

Modern tests can detect hCG levels before the time of the missed menses. Such tests can be performed in 2 minutes and are unaffected by urine contaminated by proteinuria, haematuria or bacterial contamination.

Monoclonal antibody tests for hCG and β sub-unit hCG

Sensitivity and specificity of pregnancy testing can be improved by the use of a double antibody, one being specific for the total hCG (both α and β units) and the other for the β unit hCG. The hCG is sandwiched between two antibodies, so producing agglutination and giving greater precision.

Enzyme-linked immunosorbent assays (ELISA)

ELISA tests give positive results at much lower levels of hCG and so are positive even earlier in a pregnancy. The woman can know she is pregnant by about 10 days after ovulation, i.e. before the missed period.

The mechanism is as follows:

1 The hCG is sandwiched between standard phase antibody and the enzyme-linked antibody.

2 Urine which contains hCG is added to the tube which is already coated with a double antibody.

3 Binding occurs and the enzyme, an alkaline phosphatase-linked antibody, is added. This binds with the already captured hCG.

4 A second fluid with enzyme substrate is then added; this is broken down by the bound enzymes resulting in a blue coloration.

5 A positive pregnancy test is a blue solution.

This is the basis for most commercial tests now. It does not depend upon precipitation of particles but a colour change which is always easier for the woman to spot. Many of the commercial packs include material for two tests to allow the woman to do a second check 1–2 days later to confirm the first one.

Ultrasound

Real-time ultrasound machines will detect an intrauterine gestation sac from 5 weeks of amenorrhoea, with fetal heart activity becoming visible at 6 weeks and a fetal pole visible at 7 weeks.

Transvaginal probes allow the diagnosis approximately 1 week earlier.

Antenatal visits

The current method of antenatal care was established 80 years ago and will be subject to change in the next 5 years. In particular, the visits in mid-pregnancy may be reduced.

Conventionally the woman is seen monthly from the booking visit until 28 weeks, fortnightly until 36 weeks and then weekly until delivery.

The aim of the visits is to screen the low-risk population by means of history, examination and investigation; then antenatal care for high-risk women may be carried out on a more frequent basis.

The following scheme applies to women with no obvious risk factors.

THE FIRST VISIT

Ideally the booking visit is at 8–10 weeks' gestation. More frequently now the woman's history is being taken in her own home by a community midwife.

History

1 History of maternal disease, e.g. hypertension, diabetes mellitus, tuberculosis.

2 Family history, e.g. diabetes mellitus, tuberculosis, hypertension, multiple pregnancy or the birth of a congenitally abnormal baby.

3 Establish the reliability of the LNMP (Box 2.1).

Was the woman sure of the dates?

Was the cycle regular?

Was the woman on oral contraceptives in the 2 months before she conceived?

Was there bleeding in early pregnancy?

Any of the above circumstances render the LNMP unreliable and ultrasound examination is essential to determine dates.

EXPECTED DATE OF DELIVERY (EDD)

		Example
1	Take date of 1st day of LNMP	21 September 1996
2	Take away 3 months and add a year	21 June 1997
3	Add 7 days	28 June 1997
4	This is the EDD	

Do not use if
- Dates uncertain
- Cycle not regular (i.e. outside range of 24–35 days)
- Been on oral contraception within 2 months

Box 2.1 Establishing the expected date of delivery (EDD) from the LNMP.

4 Past obstetric history. This involves listing all the pregnancies in chronological order together with the following details:

(i) Abortions and miscarriages:
   • First trimester (less than 12 weeks) or second trimester.
   • If second trimester, were they:
      (a) Relatively painless, associated with early rupture of the membranes suggesting cervical incompetence.
      (b) Associated with pain and bleeding suggestive of premature placental separation.
      (c) Associated with the delivery of a dead, macerated baby, an intrauterine death.
   • List all therapeutic abortions, their reason, gestation and method by which they were performed.

(ii) Deliveries:
   • Outcome (dead or alive).
   • Birth weight, sex and first name.
   • Gestational age.
   • Problems of the pregnancy.
   • Problems of labour and delivery.
   • Method of delivery.
   • Problems of the puerperium.
   • Problems of the newborn.
   If necessary, check these events by writing to previous hospitals.

5 Drug history. Note all drugs taken in the pregnancy so far.

6 Allergies. Note allergies to medication, food or Elastoplast.

7 Social history:
   • Detail the woman's alcohol and tobacco intake giving appropriate advice.
   • The woman's marital status, her occupation and that of her partner.
   • The living conditions and if she will have help when she returns home.

Examination

It may be that, in the absence of a relevant history and with the routine use of ultrasound, there is less need to examine the pregnant woman's pelvis. Most doctors however would still perform the following examinations:

1 Listen to the heart and take the blood pressure for a baseline reading.

2 The respiratory system.

3 The breasts to check for:
   • Lumps.

- Inverted nipples, which may require advice for breast feeding.
4   The spine for kyphosis or scoliosis.
5   The abdomen looking for scars, masses and, if the pregnancy is sufficiently advanced, the size of the uterus.
6   The legs looking for varicose veins.
7   Vaginal examination is not usually required at a booking visit but may be done:

- To confirm the pregnancy.
- To check uterine size.   } If ultrasound
- To exclude uterine or ovarian masses.   not available.
- To take a smear if the patient has not had one within the last 3 years.

Investigations

Urine

1   Proteinuria—renal disease.
2   Glucose—diabetes.
3   White blood cells—bacilluria.

Blood

1   Haemoglobin.
2   Red cell indices, particularly the mean corpuscular volume (MCV).
3   ABO and rhesus (Rh) group.
4   The presence of atypical antibodies.
5   Sickle cell screen if the patient is Afro-American.
6   Haemoglobin electrophoresis, looking for thalassaemia if the patient is Asian or Mediterranean in origin.
7   Screening test for syphilis (usually Veneral Disease Research Laboratory test). If positive, more specific tests are required.
8   Test for Australia antigen.
9   Test for rubella antibodies.
10   Human immunodeficiency virus (HIV) test. The following patients are at high risk and after appropriate counselling should be offered an HIV antibody test:

- Women from sub-Saharal Africa or women with partners from sub-Saharal Africa.
- Drug abusers or partners of drug abusers.
- Women who have bisexual partners.
- Women with haemophiliac partners.
- Women who have had a blood transfusion overseas.

11   Triple test (hCG, α-fetoprotein and oestriol) for Down's Syndrome.

Chest X-ray

Only indicated for women who have a family history of tuberculosis or who come from overseas where the disease is endemic. It is usually performed after 14 weeks' gestation.

Therapy

1   Establish a rapport between the woman and the antenatal clinic staff.

2   Show the woman where she can discover more about her pregnancy and delivery from:
- Books available.
- Mothercraft classes.
- Relaxation classes.

3   Discuss the Social Welfare benefits available.

4   Make arrangements for the medical social worker to see the woman if there are any difficulties such as care of the other children or housing.

5   Advise a visit to the dentist reasonably soon, as dental care in pregnancy is free.

6   Give dietary advice. This should be simple advice as most people in the UK have a more than adequate diet. The idea of eating for two should be discouraged and, in general, pregnant women need only an additional 500 kcal (2100 J) a day to ensure normal fetal growth.

Vegans may require specialized advice from the dietitian in order to ensure adequate nutrition throughout the pregnancy especially for certain amino acids. Similarly, some Asian women may need dietary advice or supplements of vitamin D as a consequence of living in the cloudy Northern Hemisphere.

7   Consider providing iron supplementation. The routine of prophylactic iron supplements in pregnancy is controversial. Many obstetricians only provide iron if the woman has a haemoglobin of less than 12.5 g/dl or a MCV of less than 84 fl at the booking visit. Additional reasons may be for multiple pregnancies or the last pregnancy within 2 years.

Most women's haemoglobin level will fall by about 1 g/dl due to haemodilution that occurs in pregnancy.

If iron is given, it should be taken with meals as it is only absorbed in the ferrous state and this is best achieved in the presence of vitamin C.

In the non-pregnant state, about 10% of iron is absorbed and this is thought to double in pregnancy. When supplementation is given, you should aim to give at least 100 mg of elemental iron a day. Table 2.1 lists the contents of commonly used iron tablets.

8   Vitamin supplements. These are not usually required by women receiving an adequate diet. An exception is folic acid as it is often only

CONTENT OF IRON TABLETS		
	Dose (mg)	Ferrous iron content (mg)
Ferrous sulphate (dried)	200	60
Ferrous sulphate	300	60
Ferrous fumarate	200	65
Ferrous gluconate	300	35
Ferrous succinate	100	35

Table 2.1 Dose and ferrous iron content of commonly prescribed iron tablets.

barely sufficient in many diets. The requirements in pregnancy rise from 50 μg a day to 300 μg a day. Many women are therefore given prophylactic iron tablets that also contain folic acid (500 μg a day.)

SPECIAL VISITS

Sixteen weeks: α-fetoprotein test

Neural tube defects (NTDs) account for 50% of congenital abnormalities in England and Wales. Some hospitals offer a screening programme by means of maternal serum α-fetoprotein. The test is very sensitive to gestational age and is best performed at 16 weeks' gestation checked by dating ultrasound. A positive result usually means that the woman should be referred for high-resolution ultrasound. If ths is not available, an amniocentesis may be done to determine the amniotic fluid level of α-fetoprotein. If this is high, termination is considered. Alternatively, very low α-fetoprotein levels may indicate Down's syndrome. They are taken with oestriol and hCG levels to screen for trisomy 21.

Sixteen to 20 weeks: ultrasound examination

Many hospitals in the UK now offer a routine ultrasound examination at 16–20 weeks' gestation. The aim of this ultrasound examination is:
• To establish gestational age.
• To exclude major structural abnormalities of the fetus.
• To diagnose multiple pregnancy.
• To screen for Down's Syndrome (Nuchal pad).
• To increase the bonding between the mother and the fetus.

Ultrasound uses sound at frequencies above that which can be heard by the human ear. Images are constructed from echoes that occur when ultrasound waves are reflected from boundaries between tissues or from irregularities within the tissues. A small pulse of ultrasound is sent into the tissues and a recorder in the same piece of equipment, the transducer, then detects the echoes. A high-powered computer reconstructs the echoes on a television screen to give an image of the tissues under examination. The distance between tissue boundaries can be assessed by determining the differences in time taken for the echoes to return from each boundary (Fig. 2.1).

At the 16–20-week routine ultrasound visit, the following are assessed:

• Measurement of the fetal femur length (FL) and the biparietal diameter (BPD). These measurements are used to determine the fetal age accurately (Figs 2.2 and 2.3).

• The diagnosis of a multiple pregnancy.

• The localization of the placenta. At this stage in pregnancy about 5% of women will have a placenta that is lying low in the uterus; at term, only 0.5% of women will have a real placenta praevia. Such women should be offered a rescan at 34 weeks' gestation.

• To exclude major fetal abnormalities by recognition of:

    (a) masses or cystic spaces within or attached to the fetus.

    (b) absent fetal parts, e.g. the fetal head in anencephaly.

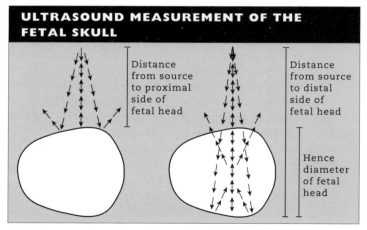

ULTRASOUND MEASUREMENT OF THE FETAL SKULL

Distance from source to proximal side of fetal head

Distance from source to distal side of fetal head

Hence diameter of fetal head

Fig. 2.1 From the combined source and receiver, the transducer, the ultrasound impulses go out in straight lines. Only those which strike reflective surfaces at right angles will return along the same path. Hence the highest and lowest points of the fetal skull may be determined. The distance between them can be measured to a sensitivity of 1 mm.

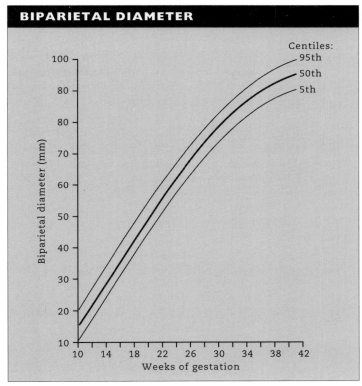

Fig. 2.2 Growth measurement of the biparietal diameter to determine the gestational age.

(c) changes in structures adjacent to the abnormality, e.g. the dilated stomach and duodenum (double bubble) seen in duodenal atresia.

(d) abnormal patterns of growth, e.g. the limbs in dwarfism.

(e) Nuchal fat pad thickens as a screen for non-structural abnormalities, e.g. Down's Syndrome.

• It is also well recognized that most women enjoy seeing ultrasound images as it increases the bonding that they feel towards their unborn infant.

LATER VISITS

If all is normal from the booking visits and the ultrasound scan session, the woman is conventionally seen as follows:

• Monthly at 20, 24, 28 and 32 weeks.

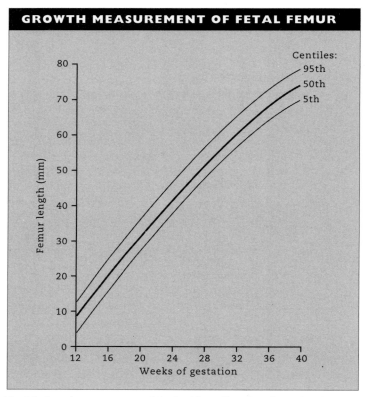

GROWTH MEASUREMENT OF FETAL FEMUR

Fig. 2.3 Growth measurement of the fetal femur length to determine the accurate gestational age.

- Fortnightly 34 and 36 weeks.
- Weekly, from 37 weeks until delivery.

At all visits

1   Check the history of recent events and at later visits ensure that the baby is moving.

2   Examine:

• Maternal weight. This is traditional and is largely for the women's benefit although excessive weight gain in late pregnancy may suggest unrecognized oedema. Fat put on in pregnancy is hard to remove afterwards.

• Blood pressure.

• The growth of the uterus and its contents.

- Test the urine for protein and glucose. This is also traditional and, in the absence of hypertension, it is less worthwhile testing for protein.

Additionally at 28 weeks

- Check the haemoglobin.
- If the woman is Rh-negative also check for the presence of Rh antibodies.
- Many now screen for gestational diabetes by doing random blood sugar at 28 weeks' gestation.

From 32 weeks onwards at all visits

- Check the lie and presentation of the fetus.

Additionally at 36 weeks

- Check haemoglobin level.
- If the patient is Rh-negative, check for the presence of antibodies.
- If the presentation is cephalic, is the head engaged?

Between 41 and 42 weeks

- Examine the cervix to assess the chances of success of induction if this is needed.

Advice to mothers

Apart from the dietary and social welfare information that should be available to the woman when she books, the following should be enquired about specifically.

Smoking

Habitual heavy smoking in pregnancy is associated with smaller babies. There is also evidence that children of heavy smokers perform less well intellectually in later life. Women should be encouraged to reduce their cigarette intake to less than five per day whilst they are pregnant or preferably to give it up. Undue pressure however should not be applied as excessive anxiety may also be harmful.

Intercourse

There is no restriction to intercourse during pregnancy unless the woman bleeds from the vagina. Mechanical problems may occur in late pregnancy so that alterations in the position of intercourse may become necessary, for example the woman may be better on top.

Alcohol

Alcohol is a cell poison to all tissues and its effects are dose related. It crosses the placenta readily and so can affect a fetus as much as an adult. Excessive drinking in pregnancy is associated with the fetal alcohol syndrome, characterized by a short nose with a low bridge, small eyes with a narrow palpebral fissure and mental retardation. Lesser degrees of alcohol intake can affect the intelligence of the child and may cause an increased incidence of mid-trimester abortion and fetal growth retardation.

No ill-effects have been described with an alcohol intake below 4 units a week.

Rest and exercise

Even in normal pregnancy, the extra weight carried by the woman may increase her sense of tiredness and lethargy. Sensible exercise such as walking and swimming or organized exericse to which the woman is accustomed (e.g. aerobics) may be allowed in pregnancy. The woman however should be advised to be sensible and to look after her body by resting when she feels tired. Many advise at least an hour's rest in the afternoon during the second half of pregnancy.

Travel

The woman should only travel over distances which are comfortable to her.

Air travel is probably better than train for long distances, but airlines can refuse to carry women over 34 weeks' gestation for international flights and over 36 weeks' gestation for domestic travel. They are the final arbiters, not the travel agents.

For long car journeys, a break every 2 hours or so should be planned, when the legs are exercised by a short walk.

Clothes

Women should be advised to wear what looks good and feels comfortable.

Maternity brassieres are often not required until late pregnancy but women should be advised to move into them as soon as they feel that their present brassiere is inadequate for support.

Shoes with flat heels should be advised during pregnancy as high heels put excessive strain on the ligaments of the back by increasing the lumbar lordosis.

Abdominal girdles are old-fashioned and have no proven value in pregnancy.

Bathing

The woman should bathe as she wishes. Avoid vaginal douching in pregnancy.

Bowels

Pregnancy tends to make women constipated because of the progestogenic effect of relaxing smooth muscles. This is best overcome by increasing fluid intake, by fresh fruit and by the use of foods rich in fibre. Laxatives should not be used unless the constipation becomes symptomatic.

Onset of labour

Many nulliparous women have no idea what to expect; up to 10% of women present with pains who are subsequently proved not to be in labour.

Advise that the onset of labour is usually accompanied by one of the following:

1 Regular painful contractions coming from the small of the back and radiating to the lower abdomen. Nulliparous women are usually advised to come into hospital when such contractions are occurring one in every 20 min.

2 A bloody or mucous show. This is not necessarily a sign of labour. If accompanied by uterine contractions women should be advised not to remain at home.

3 Rupture of the membranes accompanied by a gush of amniotic fluid. In this case, women should be advised to come to hospital immediately because of the danger of cord prolapse.

It should be emphasized that it is much better for a woman to come into hospital if she thinks she is in labour. Even if she is not, many of the causes of uterine pain may be serious and should be evaluated on the labour ward.

Psychological preparation

Pregnancy and delivery are a worry to most women. Commonly there is a fear of:

• The unknown.
• Giving birth to an abnormal baby.
• Giving birth to a dead baby.
• The pain that accompanies labour.

Many women's fears can be alleviated by proper antenatal preparation and by encouraging her to ask questions at the antenatal clinic. Women and their partners should be encouraged to attend talks about childbirth and subsequent rearing of their children. The antenatal clinic is a busy place but doctors and midwives should never appear to be rushed and should encourage women to express their fears or anxieties and to ask questions.

Psychoprophylaxis

This aims to overcome the conditioned reflex that all labours are painful. Allegedly new reflexes are taught and old ones are altered. This is supposed to raise the threshold of pain in the brain by knowledge of the situation and active participation of a neuromuscular nature. The technique attempts to reduce pain by the following:

1   Educating the patient into a fuller knowledge of what is to happen to her during labour.

2   Teaching the woman exercises to reduce cerebral activity:
   • In the first stage, slow breathing between contractions and quick shallow breathing during contractions.
   • In the transitional stage and the early second stage, women are often taught distraction therapies. They may learn a nursery rhyme and tap the rhythm of this on their chest or their partner's hand.
   • In the second stage, women are taught expulsive breathing that involves fixing the diaphragm and the upper abdomen.

To allow psychoprophylaxis to succeed, the following are required:
   • Properly trained women.
   • Properly trained doctors and midwives in the labour ward who are sympathetic to the woman's aims and know the methods involved.

Dangers
   • If the method fails and the woman requires formal analgesia, she may experience a marked sense of failure.
   • Overbreathing may lead to facial tetany by dropping CO_2 levels. This can be reversed by rebreathing using a paper bag.

Hypnotherapy

Hypnosis for pain relief in labour requires long antenatal preparation and works erratically in women. Even those who achieve deep hypnosis by conventional standards may not achieve analgesia in labour. The technique requires:
   • A skilled hypnotist who trains and conditions the woman antenatally and may have to be present in labour.
   • A susceptible patient; it is estimated that up to 90% of woman may be hypnotized, but only 50% may be susceptible to any one hypnotherapist.

Analgesia induced by successful hypnotherapy can often be remarkable and there are many reports of Caesarean sections being carried out under hypnotherapy alone.

Assessment of fetal well-being

The obstetrician is responsible for the care of two patients in labour, one of them being the fetus. The hidden patient is guarded by the following barriers:

- *Anatomical.* These can be overcome to some extent by ultrasound imaging.
- *Physiological.* These need an understanding of the interaction between fetal and maternal physiology.
- *Psychological.* These need an explanation to both the mother, her relatives, and often medical and midwifery staff to overcome the in-built resistance to investigating the unborn.

METHODS OF MEASUREMENT

Clinical

Uterine growth

In the first weeks of pregnancy this can be measured by bimanual examination. After 12 weeks' gestation it is measured by estimation of the growth of the uterine fundus, using a tape measure. Ideally these should both be performed by the same person.

Fetal growth

Once the fetus can be felt clearly after 26–28 weeks' gestation, the following can be assessed clinically:

- The size of the fetus.
- The size of the uterus.
- The amount of amniotic fluid.

Clinical assessment is at the most crude. Even in the best hands, only 40% of small babies will be recognized antenatally and, of those babies who are diagnosed to be small in the uterus, 60% will not be small at birth.

The measurement of symphyseal–fundal height

The use of a tape measure serially to monitor the height of the uterine fundus appears to be a more objective method of screening small babies than straightforward clinical palpation. Figure 2.4 shows the increase in the symphyseal–fundal height during normal pregnancy. Measurements

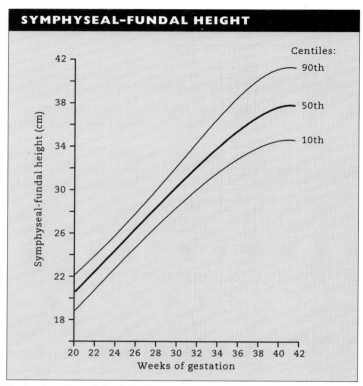

Fig. 2.4 Symphyseal–fundal height chart of a normal pregnancy.

should be plotted serially and any woman who has a low measurement should be sent for an ultrasound examination. Like all other methods, this measurement is poor at recognizing big babies.

Maternal assessment of fetal movement

This may be quantified by the following:
• The mother counts ten fetal movements entering them on a chart (Fig. 2.5). She is asked to start counting fetal movements from 9.00 a.m. and then to record the time by which she has felt ten movements. If this is later than 9.00 p.m. she is asked to report for further examination with a cardiotocograph (CTG).
• Specific hours counting. Women are asked to choose a convenient time of the day and then to count the fetal movements that occur within

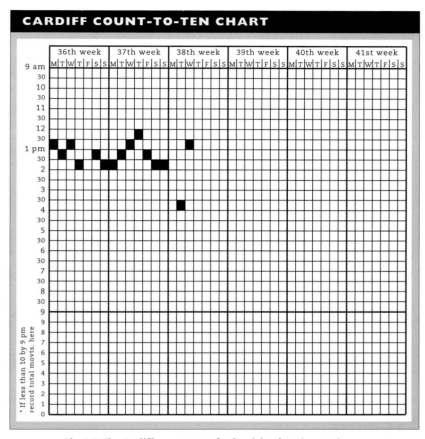

Fig. 2.5 The Cardiff count-to-ten fetal activity chart (see text).

1 hour, the same hour, every day. If there is a decline in fetal movements they are asked to report to the hospital.

Current evidence suggests that maternal appreciation of fetal movements is of value in high-risk pregnancies but does not seem to prevent unexplained stillbirths in pregnancies thought to be at low risk.

Biochemical tests

These tests have largely been replaced by biophysical methods of monitoring fetal health because of:

- A wide range of normal values obtained in pregnancy.
- The errors in laboratory measurement.

- The need, in most cases, for serial testing.
  The tests may be broadly grouped as follows:
- *Fetoplacental hormones*, e.g. oestriol. The level of oestriol in the maternal blood is dependent on interaction between steroids produced by the fetus and their conversion in the placenta.
- *Placental hormones*, e.g. human placental lactogen. The hormones are produced entirely by the placenta and may be normal even in the presence of a dead or an abnormal baby.
- *Placental proteins*. These proteins are made by the placenta or decidua and have proved to be of no greater use than human placental lactogen in monitoring late pregnancy but may be useful in early weeks.

Biophysical methods

These may be considered as:

1 Short-term methods.
  - The biophysical profile.
  - The cardiotocograph (CTG).
  - Doppler studies of the fetal circulation.

2 Medium-term methods.
  - Real-time measurements of fetal growth.
  - Doppler measurements of the uteroplacental circulation.

Short-term methods

The biophysical profile

Ultrasound examination of the following features composes the biophysical profile:

- Fetal movements.
- Fetal breathing movements.
- Fetal tone.
- The amniotic fluid volume.
- The CTG.

Each of these tests has a false-positive rate of about 20%. By combining the tests, the false-positive rate is reduced. The biophysical profile in its entirety has not become popular in the UK but aspects of it are with the CTG being the most commonly used. In addition, measurement of amniotic fluid volumes by ultrasound is often performed if the baby is found to be small.

The CTG

An antenatal record of the fetal heart rate is recorded with Doppler ultrasound. In addition, fetal movements and uterine activity are measured by an external pressure transducer. The essential features of the CTG are:

1 *The heart rate.* Between 110 and 160 beats/minute. Rates outside these limits are extremely rare antenatally.

- Baseline bradycardia usually suggests congenital heart disease.
- Fetal tachycardias are seen in the presence of anything that causes rise in the maternal pulse rate such as a maternal pyrexia. In the absence of a maternal cause, the fetal tachycardia should be taken as a sign of fetal distress.

2 *Reactivity.* In a 20-minute recording, the fetus normally produces an acceleration at least twice (Fig. 2.6). An acceleration is a rise in fetal heart rate of 15 beats/minute above the baseline that is sustained for more than 15 seconds.

The fetus is usually asleep being only awake for about 2% of the time. Fetal heart rate accelerations only occur during rapid eye movement sleep. Periods of deep sleep in fetuses should not last more than 40 minutes.

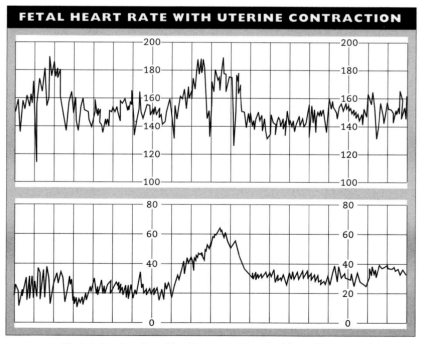

Fig. 2.6 Acceleration of fetal heart rate (above) with uterine contraction (below).

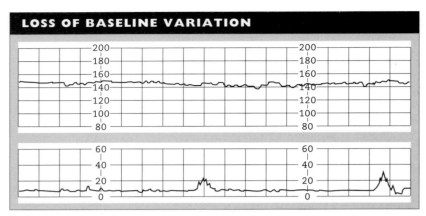

Fig. 2.7 Antenatal CTG showing loss of baseline variation.

A CTG that shows two or more accelerations in a 20 minute period is considered reactive. Non-reactive traces should not last more than 40 minutes in the third trimester.

3 *Loss of baseline variation*. (Fig. 2.7). The fetal heart rate from 26 weeks is controlled by a balance between the sympathetic and parasympathetic nervous system resulting in a natural variation of 5–15 beats/minute.

Baseline heart rate variation of less than 5 beats/minute is rarely seen antenatally although it may follow drugs such as diazepam or night sedation.

In the absence of drugs it may indicate fetal distress.

4 *Decelerations*. Antenatal decelerations in the fetal heart rate that are not associated with contractions are of serious significance and should indicate delivery taken in association with other factors.

There is no universal agreement as to how frequently the CTG should be performed. As with many other things in obstetrics, it should be planned and interpreted in the light of the woman's circumstances, e.g. if there has been a small unexplained antepartum haemorrhage (APH), only a daily CTG is required, but a growth-retarded baby in a woman with severe hypertension may warrant two or even three CTGs per day.

At present, the predictive value of a normal CTG is in doubt.

Doppler waveforms from the fetal circulation

If sound is aimed at a moving target, the echoes that return from the target will have shifted in frequency—the Doppler shift. The blood cells moving in the umbilical artery can be readily detected by Doppler ultrasound and in normal pregnancies produce the waveform shown in Fig. 2.8a.

If resistance increases in the placenta, Doppler-shifted frequencies are not recordable in the last part of diastole (absence of end-diastolic frequencies). Figure 2.8b demonstrates this phenomenon.

In a few babies, there may be a reversal of frequencies in end-diastole (Figs 2.8c and 2.9) indicating that blood which should be flowing towards

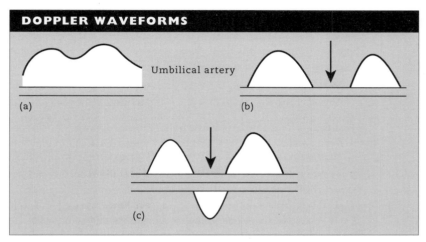

DOPPLER WAVEFORMS

Umbilical artery

(a)

(b)

(c)

Fig. 2.8 Doppler waveforms from the umbilical artery reflecting resistance to flow (impedance) in the fetal vessels of the placenta. (a) Normal. (b) Loss of end-diastolic frequencies (arrowed)—increased resistance. (c) Reversed frequencies (arrowed)—much increased resistance.

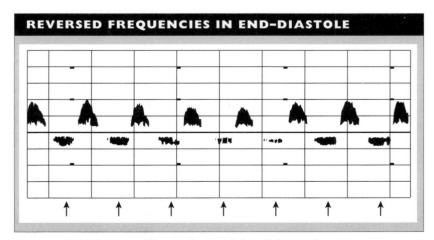

REVERSED FREQUENCIES IN END–DIASTOLE

Fig. 2.9 Reversed frequencies in end-diastole (arrowed).

the placenta for exchange O_2 and nutrients is flowing backwards towards the baby. This means that the baby will die soon.

Doppler waveforms are simple and easy to obtain and have achieved popularity over the last 5 years. Even if the baby is shown to be small on ultrasound examination, if the Doppler waveforms are normal, the outlook for the pregnancy is good.

Doppler waveforms appear to have a predictive value of about 1 week, i.e. it is unlikely that the baby will die within a week after a normal reading. Absence of end-diastolic blood flow is associated with a high incidence of both fetal hypoxia and acidosis. If not delivered, such babies have a high death rate and the survivors show an increased morbidity.

Medium-term methods

Real-time ultrasound measurements of fetal growth
Early measurement of the BPD and the FL are the most useful in establishing gestational age. Later measurements of fetal growth are best achieved by measurements of the head circumference and the abdominal circumference. Real-time ultrasound can be used to determine fetal growth in one of three ways:

1   To determine size when the fetus is thought clinically to be small.

2   As a screening test for small babies. Many hospitals now offer a second ultrasound examination at 30–34 weeks' gestation to measure the fetal abdominal circumference. If this is not low, the baby only has a small chance (approximately 10%) of being small for gestational age (SGA) at birth.

3   Serial measurements of fetal growth. Women at risk of having a SGA fetus should have serial ultrasound to document the growth velocity of their babies.

Doppler waveforms from the uteroplacental circulation
Waveforms may be recorded from the maternal uterine arteries or their first branch, the arcuate arteries. At present, the evidence is sparse but it appears that problems are associated with the depth of invasion of the placenta into the trophoplast (Fig. 2.10a) which should be complete by 22 weeks' gestation.

Failure of invasion results in a persistence of a high-resistance waveform (Fig. 2.10b) rather than the development of the usual low-resistance waveforms (Fig. 2.10a).

Women with persistently high-resistance waveforms have a high probability of developing pre-eclampsia and an asymmetrical SGA fetus.

This test looks promising and is being used more widely.

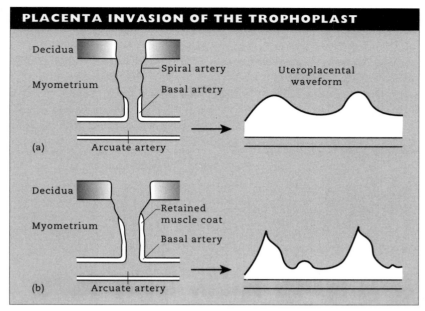

Fig. 2.10 Depth of invasion of the placenta into the trophoplast and corresponding Doppler waveforms. (a) Normal pregnancy. (b) Pre-eclampsia.

DEFINITION OF TERMS

There is much confusion in obstetric literature over the terms used to signify that the baby is small. These terms are:

• *Low birth weight (LBW)*. This term is used for a baby with a birth weight of <2500 g. This term is most useful on a worldwide basis where gestational age at delivery is often unknown. It is obvious that a baby who is <2500 g at birth may be preterm, or small, or both. Neonatal paediatricians have extended this classification to very low birth weight (VLBW) babies which indicates a birth weight of <1500 g and extremely low birth weight (ELBW) babies with a birth weight of under 1000 g.

• *Intrauterine growth retardation (IUGR)*. This is not a useful definition. IUGR is the presence of a pathology that is slowing fetal growth, which if it could be removed would allow the resumption of normal fetal growth. There are no tests available antenatally or postnatally to determine whether a baby has truly suffered from IUGR.

• *SGA*. This is a statistical definition used if the infant's birth weight is below a certain standard for the gestational age. There is no universally agreed standard and such lower limits as the tenth, the fifth, the third centile and, two standard deviations from the mean, have all been used. As the definition is statistical, one should expect for example that 10% of the normal population of babies have birth weights of less than the tenth centile. To interpret the birth weight, it is necessary to have charts derived from the local population being measured.

The term SGA is also applied antenatally when the growth or size of the fetus falls below statistically determined limits on population-derived charts.

The SGA fetus

In broad terms, impairment of fetal growth can be:
- Symmetrical SGA (Fig. 2.11). In this case the measurements of the fetal head and abdominal circumference are equally small. The baby is a miniature baby. The vast majority of these babies represent the biological lower limits of normal. Causes of symmetrical SGA are shown in Box 2.2.

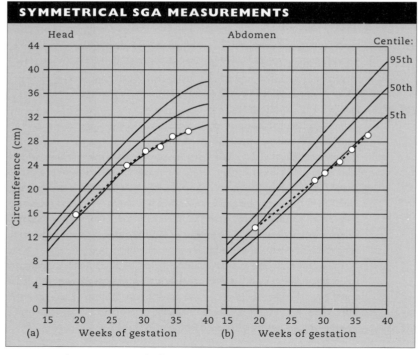

Fig. 2.11 Symmetrical SGA measurements of (a) fetal head circumference and (b) fetal abdominal circumference.

CAUSES OF SGA	
Symmetrical SGA (60%)	Asymmetrical SGA (40%)
Race (white > black > Asian)	Poor maternal response to pregnancy
Sex (boy > girl)	pre-eclampsia
Maternal size	poor trophoblast invasion
Toxins	
alcohol	
cigarettes	
heroin	
methadone	
Congenital infections	
cytomegalovirus	
parvovirus	
rubella	
syphilis	
toxoplasmosis	
Malnutrition	

Box 2.2 Causes of symmetrical growth retardation (SGA).

• Asymmetrical SGA (Fig. 2.12). This is a rarer form of impaired fetal growth, the causes of which are shown in Box 2.2. In many cases, abnormal growth is associated with absence of end-diastolic flow in the umbilical circulation. Such babies are at risk of antenatal hypoxia which may result in stillbirth, neonatal death or major mental handicap.

The differential growth patterns in these fetuses results from a redistribution of fetal blood flow. In response to underperfusion in the intervillous space, there is an increase in resistance to blood flow within the fetal circulation. This means that blood returning from the placenta to the fetus takes the path of least resistance and is diverted to the fetal brain, coronary arteries and adrenals. Initially, this is to the fetus' benefit but, if it continues for too long, then the fetal bowel, kidneys and liver become ischaemic resulting in the well-known complications of asymmetrical SGA babies, necrotizing enterocolitis, renal failure and failure of coagulation due to insufficient production of coagulation factors by the liver.

Management of SGA

Symmetrical SGA

Most of SGA fetuses represent the biological lower limits of the normal range and only require serial measurements of ultrasound growth per-

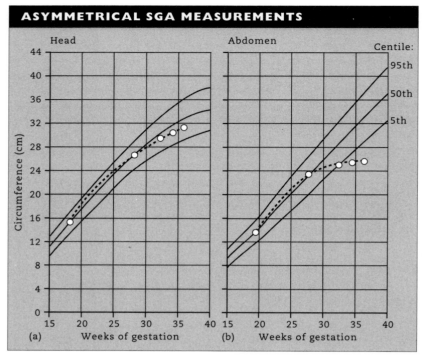

Fig. 2.12 Asymmetrical SGA measurements of (a) fetal head circumference and (b) fetal abdominal circumference.

formed on a fortnightly basis. If the baby demonstrates normal growth (see Fig. 2.11), no further action is necessary.

The only problem posed for the obstetrician is to recognize those few babies that are congenitally abnormal or infected. The following actions are recommended:

• Check maternal blood for infections that are known to cross the placenta (syphilis, toxoplasmosis, rubella, parvovirus and cytomegalovirus).
• Search the fetus carefully with ultrasound looking for structural markers that may suggest a chromosome abnormality. If these are present the baby should be karyotyped, usually by means of a fetal blood sample obtained from the umbilical cord at cordocentesis. This is of value even in the third trimester as it is well known that fetuses with trisomies are prone to fetal distress in labour. If the trisomy is lethal then after discussion with the parents a Caesarean section may not be advised should such distress develop.

Asymmetrical SGA

All fetuses show a decline in growth in the last few weeks of pregnancy (see Fig. 2.12). In some fetuses there is a cessation of abdominal growth before the reduction of the head growth and if such fetuses continue to show normal fetal circulation they are not at risk from chronic asphyxia.

Management should be:

• Fortnightly ultrasound measurements of head circumference and abdominal circumference to determine growth rate.

The amniotic fluid volume should be measured by determining the height of the largest column of fluid. This is normally between 2 and 8 cm. Less than 2 cm suggests increasing fetal compromise.

• Doppler waveforms from the umbilical circulation. If these are normal they should be repeated on a weekly basis. Delivery is not indicated in the presence of normal umbilical artery waveforms.

Absent end-diastolic flow should indicate delivery in a fetus that is considered to be viable, of greater than 28 weeks' gestation.

• In the absence of Doppler waveforms, immediate fetal well-being should be monitored by daily CTGs and maternal counting of fetal movement. Delivery is indicated for cessation of fetal growth over a 4-week period or for abnormalities of the CTG.

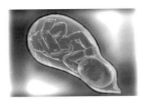

CHAPTER 3

Abnormal Conditions of Pregnancy

Nausea and vomiting in pregnancy

Early

Nausea occurs in 80% of nulliparous and 60% of multiparous women; vomiting follows in about half of these. It starts at about the time of the first missed period, worsens for 4–6 weeks and usually goes by 14–16 weeks.

Aetiology
- Reflex: stretch of peritoneum over growing uterus.
- Hormonal: rapid increase in hCG or oestrogens.
- Immunological: maternal response to fetal tissue.
- Psychological: difficult to assess but most important in the worst degrees.

Mechanism
Possibly induced through a chemosensitive trigger zone which in turn stimulates the vomiting centre. Therefore different from cause of motion sickness and so requires different treatments.

Features
- Is not usually accompanied by long periods of nausea.
- Does not cause constitutional upset.
- About a third of cases do not occur in the morning.

Management
- Exclude specific causes: urinary infection or reaction to iron tablets.

- Rest: if morning sickness, stay in bed until having eaten.
- Frequent small, unrich meals.
- Drugs:

Antihistamines	Phenergan ⎱	good but make women
	Anthisan ⎬	sleepy. Therefore do not
	Promethazine ⎰	use if still working.
Dopamine antagonists	Metoclopramide	
Tranquillizers	prochlorperazine (5 mg tds).	

- Give advice that the condition is self-limiting.

Late

Occasional vomiting in last few weeks; due to:

1 Mass in abdomen pushing up stomach.
2 Small hiatus hernia or oesophageal reflux.
   Can be treated with:
1 Antacids and gastric-coating agents.
2 Posture advice to reduce effects of reflux.

Labour

Very common; due to:

1 Pressure factors mentioned above.
2 Work of labour.
3 Drugs given for pain relief:
   - 25% of women will vomit when given morphine.
   - 15% of women will vomit when given pethidine.

   Therefore always combine an antihistamine with pain relief, e.g. pethi-dine 100 mg + Phenergan 25 mg. (Beware hypotensive effects of repeating these combinations.)

Hyperemesis gravidarum

Incidence

Less than 1 : 1000 pregnancies in UK; a rare condition in the endogenous population.

Aetiology

As with early vomiting, but there is often much greater emphasis on psychological factors (e.g. fear of loss of job, fear of labour, rejection of pregnancy).

Progress

Can lead to:

- Dehydration.
- Hypovolaemia.
- Electrolyte depletion.
- Vitamin deficiency, particularly thiamine.
- Death from liver failure or the end processes of the above.

Presentation
- Cannot retain food or fluid.
- Weight loss because loss of body fluid and burning up of fat.
- Haemoconcentration and unstable acid–base balance.
- Ketosis.

Management
1   Exclude other diseases:
- Urinary infection.
- Hiatus hernia and gall bladder disease.
- Obstructive gut lesions.
- CNS-expanding lesions.
2   Exclude obstetric cause:
- Multiple pregnancy.
- Hydatidiform mole.
- Acute yellow atrophy of the liver.
3   Restore fluid and electrolyte balance intravenously (i.v.).
4   Administer vitamins i.v., especially B group.
5   Specific anti-vomiting drugs, e.g. Ancoloxin or Maxolon.
6   Psychological treatment—most respond to suggestion. If not, formal psychotherapy is needed.
7   Therapeutic abortion—very rarely required.

Pre-eclampsia

Pre-eclampsia (pregnancy-induced hypertension) is a disorder is specific to pregnancy. It carries the following risks to the mother and fetus:
1   *The mother*
- Cerebrovascular accident.
- Renal failure.
- Heart failure.
- Coagulation failure.
- Liver failure.
- Adrenal failure.
- Eclampsia: a generalized convulsive disorder like epilepsy but which is peculiar to pregnancy.

2 *The fetus*
- Asymmetrical growth retardation.
- Placental abruption.
- Iatrogenic preterm delivery.

Definitions

The currently internationally agreed definitions of hypertensive disease in pregnancy are:
- Pregnancy-induced hypertension (PIH): hypertension occurring for the first time after 20 weeks' gestation.
- Pregnancy-associated hypertension (PAH): hypertension occurring before pregnancy or during the first 20 weeks.
- PAH with superimposed PIH.

Hypertension in pregnancy is defined as one of the following:
- Blood pressure of 140/90 mmHg on two occasions more than 4 hours apart.
- A rise of more than 30 mmHg in systolic blood pressure over the booking blood pressure.
- A rise in more than 20 mmHg in diastolic blood pressure over the booking figure.

PIH may be classified as:
- *Mild*: a blood pressure of less than 140/100 mmHg without proteinuria.
- *Moderate*: a blood pressure of less than 160/110 mmHg without proteinuria.
- *Severe*: a blood pressure of more than 160/110 mmHg; and the presence of proteinuria.

Proteinuria in pregnancy is defined as the following:
- More than 300 mg/l on a 24-hour collection of urine.

Many older texts in obstetrics classify pre-eclampsia as two of the three following symptoms:
- Hypertension.
- Proteinuria.
- Oedema.

This is not now used for several reasons:
- Oedema occurs in more than 40% of all pregnancies. In the absence of hypertension, it is usually associated with slightly heavier babies.
- The combination of oedema and proteinuria without hypertension is more suggestive of underlying renal disease.
- Hence oedema is no longer considered important, nor is excessive weight gain necessarily a measure of severity.

Prevalence

This varies with the population but in the UK 10–15% of primigravid women will develop some form of hypertension. Of these, about 6% may be considered as suffering from pregnancy-induced hypertension and 2% will develop the more severe form associated with proteinuria.

PIH is almost entirely a disease of primigravidae. It only occurs in multigravid women under the following conditions:
- Those who have had it severely in the first pregnancy.
- Those who have changed their partner between pregnancies.
- Pregnancies complicated by hydatidiform mole.
- Multiple pregnancies.

Aetiology

The precise mechanism is unknown; the following are recognized:
- Women who develop pre-eclampsia have a failure of the second wave of trophoblastic invasion (Fig. 3.1; see also Fig. 2.11b).
- This failure probably leads to a local alteration of the prostacyclin : thromboxane ratio. Both these prostaglandins are produced by trophoblast and exert opposite effects (Fig. 3.1). In PIH, the balance of the ratio appears to favour thromboxane. This leads to local vasoconstriction and platelet agglutination on already damaged vessels.
- The combination of the above two factors is associated with failure of the initial fall in peripheral resistance and hence blood pressure in mid-pregnancy is maintained — it normally shows a marked fall. Subsequent narrowing or clotting of the abnormal blood vessels leads to a further increase in peripheral resistance and hence hypertension.
- The narrowing of the blood vessels also leads to decreased perfusion of the intervillous space and hence the development of an asymmetrical SGA fetus.
- In severe disease there is also development of immune complexes which are deposited on the basement membrane of the kidneys. The mechanisms of PIH are summarized in Fig. 3.1. It is not clear as to why the second wave of trophoblastic invasion should fail in some women.

Clinical course

Fulminating disease

Fulmination is a rise in blood pressure associated with the signs and symptoms of impending eclampsia. It is an obstetric emergency and failure to start prompt treatment may lead to eclampsia or a maternal cerebrovascular accident.

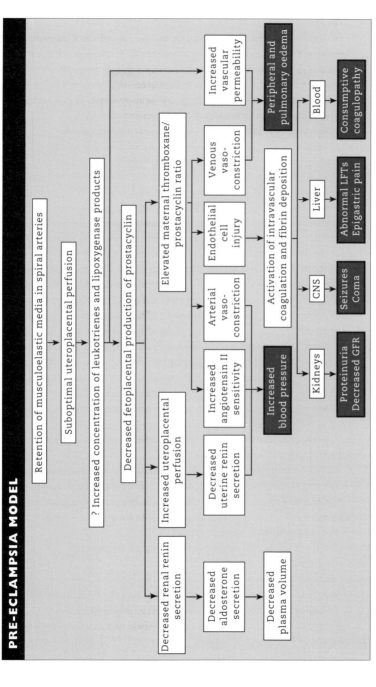

Fig. 3.1 Proposed model to explain pre-eclampsia; tinted boxes are the manifestations. CNS = central nervous system; GFR = glomerular filtration rate; LFT = liver function test.

Symptoms

- *Frontal and often occipital headache* due to cerebral oedema. The headache is dragging or throbbing in nature and is worse when the woman is supine. It occurs classically first thing in the morning and resolves to some extent during the day if the patient is mobile.
- *Visual disturbances* due to oedema of the optic nerve or the retina consisting of black holes in the visual field (scotomata).
- *Epigastric pain.* This is due to stretching of the liver capsule.

Signs

- *Hyper-reflexia and clonus.* This is due to the cerebral oedema and gives the clinical picture of an upper motor neuron lesion.

    Hyper-reflexia, in obstetric terms, is defined as the ability to obtain the reflex away from the tendon that usually causes it, e.g. the knee jerk reflex occurs by tapping the anterior surface of the tibia rather than the infrapatellar tendon.

    Clonus in obstetric terms is only considered serious if it is sustained for more than six beats.
- *A rapid rise in blood pressure.*

Treatment

The disease process starts to reverse as soon as the placenta is delivered and hence the solution to fulminating pre-eclampsia is to end the pregnancy. Before this happens, the maternal condition must be prevented from worsening:

- Aspirin has been used prophylactically to prevent or lessen the severity of pre-eclampsia. It does not work.
- Control the maternal blood pressure. At present this is done by the use of i.v. hydralazine or labetalol.
- Prevent maternal fits with i.v. diazepam or magnesium sulphate.

    Having controlled the blood pressure, the baby should be delivered. The aim is to deliver the baby vaginally but indications for Caesarean section are:

- An unripe cervix.
- An abnormal fetal position such as a breech presentation.
- Fetal distress.
- Abruption of the placenta.
- A failed induction.
- Difficulty in controlling the maternal blood pressure.

Moderate disease

All primigravidae who have a sustained blood pressure of 140/90 mmHg or more should be monitored in a fetal day centre or in hospital as the subsequent course of their disease cannot be predicted. In the absence of fulminating hypertension, the following management features are relevant.

Maternal

I   *4-hourly measurement of blood pressure.* There is no evidence that treating maternal blood pressure with antihypertensive drugs alters the course of the pre-eclamptic disease process or improves the prognosis of the fetus, but treatment is indicated if the maternal circulation is threatened. Sustained blood pressures of more than 160/110 mmHg would therefore indicate treatment, unless delivery was imminent. The current choice of therapy is oral methyldopa or labetalol but magnesium sulphate is often helpful.

2   *Assessment of maternal renal function.* On admission, all patients should have:

- Plasma urea and electrolyte estimation.
- Plasma urate levels.
- Twice-weekly measurements of creatinine clearance and total urinary protein excretion.

A severe fall in creatinine clearance to levels of less than 40 ml/minute or a rise in urate would probably be an indication for the delivery.

Fetal well-being

- Real-time ultrasound assessment of fetal size. If this indicates asymmetrical SGA then carry out:
    (a)   daily or twice daily CTGs;
    (b)   a weekly examination of the umbilical circulation by Doppler ultrasound.
- Doppler waveforms from uteroplacental circulation.
    In moderate disease, delivery is indicated for:
- Fulmination.
- Declining maternal renal function.
- Fetal distress, which usually means an abnormal CTG or absence of end-diastolic flow in the Doppler measurement of the umbilical circulation.
- Placental abruption.
    In the absence of the above features, most obstetricians would consider inducing the pregnancy after 34 weeks' gestation, if the cervix is favourable and neonatal facilities are adequate.

Mild disease

Women with mild PIH may be discharged from hospital and assessed as outpatients if:

- The blood pressure remains below 140/100 mmHg.
- There is no significant proteinuria.
- The fetus does not demonstrate asymmetrical SGA.

The woman's blood pressure should be monitored at least twice a week and fetal growth should be monitored fortnightly by ultrasound. If the condition does not deteriorate, it is difficult to justify induction of labour although few obstetricians would be prepared to let these women go past 40 weeks' gestation.

Prognosis

Maternal

In the absence of eclampsia, maternal mortality should be low, but it must be remembered that PIH is one of the leading factors of maternal death, even in developed countries. Maternal morbidity may occur from subsequently badly managed fluid balance.

If the woman can be helped over the first 48 hours after delivery without serious injury, then the disease usually rapidly gets better. This is usually indicated by a diuresis and there is no permanent long-term renal or vascular damage in women with PIH.

Fetal

The perinatal mortality rate (PNMR) increases with the severity of the disease, but may be summarized as follows:

- Mild: no change in PNMR.
- Moderate: slightly increased depending upon gestation at birth.
- Severe: double PNMR.
- Severe PIH superimposed on PAH: treble PNMR.

The morbidity to the baby is difficult to quantify as it depends upon the gestation at delivery and the fetal size.

Eclampsia

Eclampsia is characterized by epileptiform fits associated with hypertension of a moderate to severe degree. In the UK it is rare with a prevalence of about 1:3000 deliveries. Worldwide it is usually preceded by pre-eclampsia, but the quality of antenatal care in the UK now is such that three-quarters of cases of eclampsia occur without pre-existing evidence of hypertension.

Prevalence

In the UK the disease is rare because of:

1   Better antenatal care which has led to earlier recognition of pre-eclampsia.

2   More aggressive treatment of pre-eclampsia which has lessened the incidence of subsequent eclampsia.

- The rate of eclampsia may be taken as a guide to antenatal care—to its availability, usage and quality.
- Less than 1% of women in the UK with moderate or severe PIH will go on to develop eclampsia.

Aetiology

- Cerebral oedema.
- Cerebral vasoconstriction.
- Cerebral hypoxia.

These lead to cerebral ischaemia and hence fits.

Clinical course

At present in the UK about 25% of women with eclampsia will have a fit before labour; most of the rest are likely to have a fit in the postpartum period. The character of the fit is very similar to an epileptic fit with a typical fit consisting of:

- Twitching: 30 seconds.
- Tonic phase: 30 seconds.
- Clonic phase: 2 minutes.
- Coma: 10–30 minutes.

Such fits may repeat frequently.

Treatment

Aims

- Keep the woman alive during the fit.
- Prevent more fits.
- Terminate the pregnancy.

Prevention

- Magnesium sulphate may reduce incidence and severity of fits. It is used widely in the US but not yet in the UK.

During the fit

- Turn the woman on her side.
- Maintain the airway.
- Stop the fit by giving i.v. diazepam or magnesium sulphate.

After the fit
- Prevent further fits. This is usually done by giving a continuous infusion of diazepam or intramuscular magnesium sulphate.
- If the woman is not in hospital, arrange an emergency transfer giving adequate anticonvulsants to cover the journey.
- Lower the blood pressure by use of i.v. hydralazine or labetalol.
- Deliver the baby. As with fulminating PIH, such women are best if the baby is delivered vaginally, as this speeds the recovery process. The indications for Caesarean section are those listed in the section on fulminating PIH.

Prognosis

Maternal mortality
In the UK death from eclampsia is rare with the woman more likely to die from the hypertensive effects on the cerebral circulation from a cerebro-vascular accident.

Fetal mortality
The risk of the fetus dying during an eclamptic fit is about 300/1000. Overall, the perinatal mortality from eclampsia is of the order of 150/1000 deliveries due mostly to intrauterine death from hypoxia or neonatal death from prematurity.

Rhesus incompatibility

RH GENES

The Rh genes are carried on a pair of chromosomes. There are six Rh antigens (*C, D, E, c, d, e*) of which *D* and *d* are the most important, for upon these depend whether a person is designated Rh-positive or Rh-negative.

The individual making these gametes may be heterozygous if some of the gametes contain *c, d, e* and others *C, D, E*, or the person may be homozygous if all gametes are *c, d, e*.

Thus:

$$\left.\begin{array}{cc} c & c \\ d & d \\ e & e \end{array}\right\}$$ is the make up of a Rh-negative person.

$$\left.\begin{array}{cc|cc} C & C & C & c \\ D & d & \text{or} \quad D & d \\ e & e & e & e \end{array}\right\}$$ is a Rh-positive person who is heterozygous.

$$\left. \begin{array}{cc} C & C \\ D & D \\ e & e \end{array} \quad \mathrm{or} \quad \begin{array}{cc} C & c \\ D & D \\ e & E \end{array} \right\} \text{ is a Rh-positive person who is homozygous.}$$

There is no problem if the woman is Rh-positive, even if her partner is an Rh-negative man; if homozygous, all her children will be Rh-positive; if heterozygous, she may have an Rh-negative child but that is no problem.

Should she be Rh-negative and her partner homozygous Rh-positive (35% of the male population), she will always have an Rh-positive child.

He may be heterozygous Rh-positive (65% of the male population) producing equal numbers of Rh-positive and Rh-negative gametes. He has equal chances of giving his Rh-negative partner an Rh-positive or an Rh-negative child.

The genotypes are not equally distributed in the population. In UK the commonest are the 85% of Rh-positive people

$$\begin{array}{llll}
\begin{array}{cc} C & c \\ D & d \\ e & e \end{array} \; 30\% &
\begin{array}{cc} c & C \\ D & D \\ e & e \end{array} \; 20\% &
\begin{array}{cc} C & C \\ D & D \\ e & e \end{array} \; 10\% &
\begin{array}{cc} c & c \\ D & d \\ E & e \end{array} \; 10\%
\end{array}$$

(*D* is present in all the common genotypes);

and the 15% Rh-negative

$$\begin{array}{cc} c & C \\ d & d \\ e & e. \end{array}$$

IMMUNIZATION

An Rh-positive mother cannot be immunized against the Rh factor and so there are no problems for her and her baby.

The Rh-negative woman can be affected if she is inoculated with Rh-positive blood. The Rh group antigens evoke an antibody response; antibodies against the Rh group (most marked against the D antigen) will be made in the mother's reticuloendothelial system.

In Rh-negative women, the inoculation of Rh-positive cells can occur:

1 In an incompletely crossmatched transfusion.

2 During the transplacental passage of red cells from an Rh-positive baby.

The latter is more likely in a major fetomaternal bleed occurring in an APH, spontaneous or therapeutic abortion, amniocentesis, after an external cephalic version (ECV) or, most commonly, in labour when the transplacental passage of red cells occurs in the third stage, when the placenta is being squeezed and massaged by the uterus.

In most Rh-incompatible pregnancies no antibody is formed until after the first fetomaternal bleed most commonly in the third stage of labour and, consequently, the baby of the first pregnancy is unaffected.

In subsequent pregnancies, if the fetus is Rh-positive, small fetomaternal bleeds may have evoked a major secondary antibody response in a sensitized woman. Large amounts of antibody (immunoglobulin G (IgG)) cross the placenta and can cause increasingly severe Rh disease in successive pregnancies if the fetus is Rh-positive. The antibody weakens the envelopes of the fetal red cells, which are then broken down in the spleen. Depending on the speed and degree of cell breakdown, this can produce:

1   Fetal anaemia.

2   Hyperbilirubinaemia. *In utero* the excess bilirubin is removed across the placenta to the maternal circulation. Following delivery the bilirubin accumulates and so the infant becomes jaundiced.

3   Oedema.

Clinical picture

This can vary.

•   The fetus may die *in utero* if the anaemia is severe enough.

•   The infant may be born grossly anaemic and oedematous with hepato-splenomegaly — hydrops fetalis. There is a rapid rise in bilirubin following birth for *in utero* the excess bilirubin has been removed by the placenta. Jaundice develops rapidly within the first 24 hours of life.

•   The infant can be anaemic and continues to break down red blood cells after delivery as the maternal Rh antibodies are still circulating in his blood and so can become more anaemic and jaundiced during the postnatal period.

Management

Prevent

Either:

Give 500 i.u. anti-*D* immunoglobulin to all Rh negative women at 28 and 36 weeks;

or:

Be selective and give 250 i.u. anti-*D* immunoglobulin:

•   After therapeutic abortion.

•   After spontaneous abortion.

•   After amniocentesis.

•   Give 500 i.u. units.

•   After ECV.

- After delivery of any Rh-positive baby especially if that baby is ABO-compatible. This measure has reduced the effects of Rh disease enormously in Western society.
- Use a Kleihauer's test to indicate the worst affected (i.e. needing a second dose of anti-D immunoglobulin).

Detect at-risk fetus
- Maternal Rh screening, anti-D antibody titres.
- Serial ultrasound examinations for fetal oedema.
- Amniocentesis and optical density of fluid.
- Check cord blood.

History
1 Check history of:
  - Previous transfusion.
  - Jaundiced babies.
  - Exchange transfusions.
  - Hydrops.
  - Stillbirth or neonatal death.

2 Check all Rh-negative pregnant women for albumin antibodies and, if above 20 i.u./l, perform an indirect Coombs' test.
Check:
- On booking.
- If negative at booking, at 24, 28 and 34 weeks.
- If positive at booking, at 20, 24, 28, 32 and 36 weeks or more frequently if rapidly rising.

If antibody titre rises above 1 : 8 by 20 weeks, do an amniocentesis.

To reduce risks carry out amniocentesis under ultrasound guidance using a 20 gauge needle. Remove 5–10 ml of amniotic fluid. Check optical density. Compare with Lilley's at-risk graph (Fig. 3.2).

3 Check cord blood immediately after birth for:
  - ABO group and Rh group.
  - Hb.
  - Direct Coombs' test.
  - Bilirubin.

Treat
- Intrauterine transfusion.
- Elect time of delivery.
- Exchange transfusion after delivery.
- Phototherapy after delivery.
- Top-up transfusion.

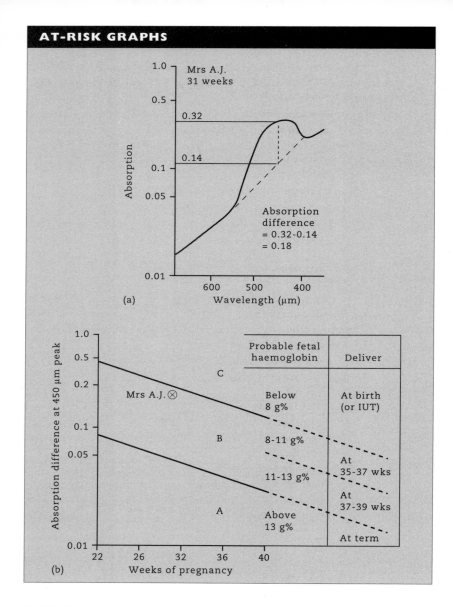

Fig. 3.2 At-risk graphs. (a) Spectral absorption curve of amniotic fluid in haemolytic disease. The peak, found at 450 μm, is measured from a line joining the beginning and ending curves. The absorption difference represents the amount of bilirubin breakdown products. (b) Probability of risk chart. It shows the height of the peak of pigment in amniotic fluid at different maturities of pregnancy. Zone C is severely affected, B moderately, and A slightly affected. IUT = intrauterine transfusion.

Intrauterine transfusion

In very severe Rh disease the fetus can die *in utero* from anaemia and hydrops before he can be delivered. An intrauterine transfusion can prolong the life *in utero* of an infant to a gestation where the risks of prematurity are estimated as being less than those of the Rh disease. This can be done by an:

1 Intraperitoneal transfusion.
2 Umbilical vein transfusion guided by ultrasound.

Rh-negative blood is either transfused under ultrasound control into the fetal peritoneal cavity, or into an umbilical vein. Repeat as necessary, according to amniotic optical density, or fetal haematocrit. The intravenous route is becoming increasingly the preferred method.

Choose time of induction and best method of delivery

Balance the risks of prematurity (too soon) with that of worsening Rh disease (too late). Consider the risks of vaginal delivery and be prepared for a lower segment Caesarean section (LSCS). The paediatric team should be in close liaison and a senior paediatrician present at the delivery with fresh Rh-negative blood.

Resuscitation and exchange transfusion

Good resuscitation is essential. In an anaemic and premature infant, lung disease is common. It can be due to:

• Surfactant deficiency at very early delivery.
• Pulmonary oedema from anaemia and hypoproteinaemia.
• Hypoplastic lungs secondary to pleural effusions.

In severe Rh haemolytic disease of the newborn, an umbilical artery catheter should be inserted as soon as possible to assess and control PaO_2 and pH.

• Central venous pressure should be measured.
• Drain pleural effusions and ascites at resuscitation.

Indications for exchange transfusion
Early: Decision mainly based on cord Hb (in addition consider history of previously affected babies).

1 Cord Hb < 12 g/dl.
2 Strongly positive Coombs' test.
3 Cord bilirubin > 85 μmol/l.

Late: Usually done for hyperbilirubinaemia. Serum bilirubin should be measured at least 4-hourly from birth. Watch for rapidly rising bilirubin. Level at which to do an exchange transfusion depends on gestation and condition of infant. Record bilirubin measurements on graph and estimate time when bilirubin will reach certain preset value, e.g. in 1-kg well infant, 200 µmol/l; or, in 3-kg well infant, 350 µmol/l. Do an exchange transfusion when bilirubin just below preset level.

Aims
- Treats anaemia.
- Washes out IgG antibodies.
- Decreases degree of haemolysis.
- Removes bilirubin.
- Prevents kernicterus.

Continuous phototherapy
For jaundice from birth, until bilirubin falling.

Top-up transfusion
A late anaemia can develop. If haemoglobin falls below 7 g/dl, give top-up transfusion. Prophylactic oral folate will be required.

Genital tract bleeding in early pregnancy

MISCARRIAGE OR ABORTION
Abortion is the expulsion of a dead fetus before 24 weeks' gestation. The word may imply motivation to the public although most abortions are spontaneous; it is better to use the word miscarriage.

Prevalence
25% of clinically apparent pregnancies miscarry before 12 weeks.

Threatened miscarriage
This is characterized by painless bleeding in early pregnancy. On examination:
- The cervical internal os is usually closed.
- The uterus is compatible with the gestational age.

Treatment
Ultrasound will show a live fetus; this is the best predictor of an on-going pregnancy. If the fetus is still alive following the acute bleed, the survival rate is approximately 85%. There is no evidence that these women benefit from hospital admission or bed rest; they should be allowed home. It is probably prudent to advise them to avoid intercourse, although there is no scientific basis for this.

Inevitable miscarriage

This is characterized by pain, bleeding, the passage of clots and sometimes the products of conception. If, on examination, the internal os is open, the miscarriage has either happened or is bound to happen. They are sub-classified as:

• *Complete*: all the products of conception have been expelled. This may happen after 16 weeks of amenorrhoea, but rarely before.

• *Incomplete*. Some or all of the products of conception remain and there is a substantial risk of continuing bleeding.

Treatment

At risk for:

• Continuing haemorrhage.
• Give syntometrine.
• Sepsis.

    Evacuation of retained products of conception (ERPC) should be arranged under general anaesthetic as soon as possible. If the woman is Rh-negative she should receive 250 i.u. of anti-*D* immuno-globulin.

Missed miscarriage

This is often difficult to differentiate from a threatened miscarriage except where the uterus shows a marked discrepancy from that expected from the woman's LNMP. Ultrasound will show the absence of a fetus who has died earlier in pregnancy.

Treatment

Most need an evacuation of the retained products of conception. There is a theoretical risk of a clotting abnormality, but it is rare unless the fetus has been dead for 3–4 weeks and is not a problem in clinical practice for first trimester abortions.

Septic miscarriage

The woman presents with systemic symptoms including pyrexia and general feelings of being unwell. On examination, the uterus is tender and there may be an offensive discharge.

Treatment

An urgent evacuation of retained products of conception under antibiotic cover is needed. Most obstetricians now practise:

• High-dose broad-spectrum i.v. antibiotics immediately before the operation to cover the bacteraemia that might follow the ERPC.

- ERPC by a senior experienced obstetrician. When the uterus is septic and pregnant, it is very easy to perforate.
- Careful follow-up for the woman with 4-hourly measurements of pulse and temperature.
- If the woman still remains pyrexial after 48 hours of appropriate antibiotics, then it is usual to add in i.v. heparin because she may have septic thrombi in the pelvic veins.
- Observe for septic shock.

Management

Women who bleed in early pregnancy should have speculum examination to check the cervix. If the internal os is open, then the pregnancy is lost and there is little role for ultrasound examination. Women in whom the cervical os is closed should have an ultrasound examination as soon as possible.

Ultrasound examination for bleeding in early pregnancy is of value:

- In pregnancies that are more than 6–7 weeks' gestation, fetal heart activity and a fetal pole should be visualized.
- Incomplete miscarriages show no evidence of a normal gestation and often only a few remaining products of conception are seen in the cavity.
- A missed miscarriage may be diagnosed with an abdominal scan after 7 weeks' gestation. At this stage, an empty sac (Fig. 3.3) is seen with no evidence of fetal activity. Experienced ultrasonographers can make the diagnosis from one examination but, if there is doubt, a rescan a week later

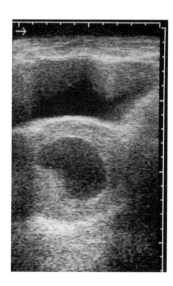

Fig. 3.3 Ultrasound scan showing a missed miscarriage after 7 weeks' gestation.

will clarify the situation. In a normal pregnancy, the volume of the gestational sac will have doubled in size, and the fetus will become visible.

• Ultrasound will also diagnose rare causes of bleeding in early pregnancy such as a hydatidiform mole.

Recurrent spontaneous miscarriage (RSM)

This is defined as the loss of three or more consecutive pregnancies before 20 weeks' gestation. It is usually classified as:

1 *Primary*: three or more consecutive miscarriages without a term pregnancy.

2 *Secondary*: three or more consecutive miscarriages following a term pregnancy.

Prevalence

About 1% of women, a figure that is higher than expected by chance.

Prognosis

The chances of successful pregnancy following three previous miscarriages (RSM) are about 60%; this figure is high enough for many obstetricians to question that any treatment is justified. Understandably however, couples often do not share this opinion.

The single most important predictive factor for miscarriage is the woman's previous obstetric history. Women with a history of successful pregnancy rarely miscarry.

Causes

• Chromosome translocation in the parents.
• Maternal diabetes mellitus.
• Maternal thyroid disease.
• Genital tract infections.
• Systemic lupus erythematosus.
• Women with polycystic ovaries.
• Women with an arcuate or subseptate uterus.
• There is little evidence of an immunological basis for RSM. Although the theories are attractive, clinical trials generally do not support an increase in successful pregnancy rates after maternal immunization with paternal leucocytes, with pooled lymphocytes or with trophoblast extracts.

ECTOPIC PREGNANCY

This is pregnancy implanted outside the cavity of the uterus (Fig. 3.4).

Women at higher risk include those:

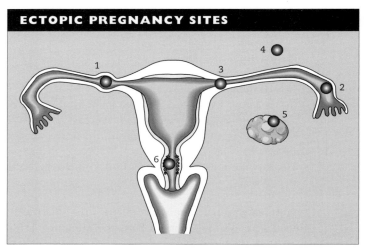

Fig. 3.4 Sites for ectopic pregnancies. 1, Fallopian tube—isthmial; 2, Fallopian tube—ampullary; 3, cornual; 4, abdominal; 5, ovarian; 6, cervical.

- With previous salpingitis.
- With a previous ectopic pregnancy.
- Who ovulate late in the cycle.
- With previous tubal surgery.
- On progesterone-only pill.
- With IUD.

Incidence
Depends on the population. In the UK 1 : 200 pregnancies, nearly all in the Fallopian tube.

Isthmial
Medial two-thirds of tube. Wall cannot stretch, therefore early rupture (4–8 weeks' gestation).

Symptoms
Sudden acute lower abdominal pain. May occur before any amenorrhoea noticed.

Signs
- Shock.
- Rigid abdomen.

- Very tender uterus and too guarded to tell details of adnexa in vaginal examination.

Treatment

Conventional
Resuscitate with blood and operate immediately. Do not await full correction of hypovolaemia before starting surgery. Clamp off bleeding area. Then carry out either a partial salpingectomy (leaving ampullary end for possible later reanastomosis) or a total salpingectomy. In either case try to conserve ovarian tissue.

Laparoscopic
Some experienced laparoscopists will treat a bleeding ectopic by endoscopy with coagulation or loop ligature of the tube. This is only for the proficient operators.

Ampullary

Lateral third of tube. More stretch allowed by laxer muscle wall, therefore later onset of symptoms (8–12 weeks' gestation). Nearer lateral ostium and so blood may leak at lower pressure to peritoneal cavity.

Symptoms
Intermittent, dull, vague pains in hypogastrium over several days.

Signs
Tender uterus and pouch of Douglas with boggy adnexal mass.

Management
Make the diagnosis:
1 hCG level raised.
2 Ultrasound:
   - Empty uterus.
   - Thickened decidua.
   - Fluid in pouch of Douglas.
   - May see ectopic gestational sac (do not expect this).
3 Laparoscopy.

Treatment
At laparoscopy:
1 Inject fetotoxic drug into unruptured ectopic pregnancy, e.g. methotrexate.

2   Suck conceptus out of lateral end of tube.

3   Incise tube for 2 cm on antimesenteric border over conceptus; remove and close tube with two or three fine Prolene sutures.

4   Partial salpingectomy conserving ovary.

Whilst partial or total excision of tube and conceptus was conventional treatment, laparoscopic methods are being used more widely now.

HYDATIDIFORM MOLE

A benign tumour of the trophoblast; the malignant extension is choriocarcinoma.

Incidence

1 : 2000 pregnancies in the West and much commoner in the Far East.

Causes

An absence of central blood vessels in the villus prevents exchange and so the embryo dies. The villi which survive become swollen, distended with fluid, and resemble a bunch of small grapes.

Most hydatidiform moles are homozygous with a 46, XX karyotype. This probably follows fertilization of an oocyte by duplicated haploid sperm or parthenogenesis.

Presentation—history

1   Uterine bleeding without pain in the first weeks of pregnancy.

2   Feeling unwell.

3   Excessive sickness.

4   Passage of vesicles like small grapes less than 1 cm. This is unusual.

Examination

1   Uterus may be larger than the period of gestation, if gestation is advanced beyond 14 weeks, otherwise the uterus is the expected size or even smaller.

2   If uterus is large enough to palpate distinctly, soft boggy feel.

3   Fetal heart cannot be detected and fetal parts not felt.

4   Raised blood pressure may be present early in pregnancy (because of concomitant early pre-eclampsia).

5   Bilateral ovarian luteal cysts may be felt.

Investigations

1   An ultrasound scan shows no fetal echoes but diffuse multiple cysts like light shining through the coarse foam of a bubble bath (Fig. 3.5).

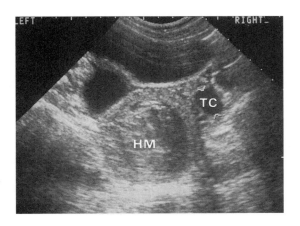

Fig. 3.5 Ultrasound scan of a hydatidiform mole (HM) with a theca-luteal cyst (TC) in the ovary.

2 Serum and urinary hCG levels rise in normal pregnancy to a maximum at about 16 weeks (Fig. 3.6). In a hydatidiform mole these levels rise very much more rapidly and to much higher levels.

Management

The blood loss can be heavy and so first treatment must be in preventing or reducing haemorrhage.

1 Admit to hospital; give Syntocinon if bleeding.

2 Put up i.v. oxytocin to make uterus contract.

3 Correct blood loss.

4 Anaesthetize and remove vesicles by vacuum extraction through the cervix, which rarely requires any dilatation. Send specimen to laboratory to exclude choriocarcinoma.

5 Watch for bleeding after delivery and be prepared to increase oxytocic drugs.

6 Arrange follow-up in conjunction with one of the regional centres for trophoblast disease (Charing Cross Hospital, London; Jessop Hospital, Sheffield; or Ninewell's Hospital, Aberdeen).

7 Provide proper contraceptive advice to prevent pregnancy for 1 year.

Prognosis

Usually good. Some 10% develop trophoblastic malignancy (choriocarcinoma). All women with a hydatidiform mole are followed for 2 years with estimations of hCG monthly for 6 months and 3-monthly for 2 years. If the hCG level does not fall within 6 weeks, treatment with methotrexate or actinomycin D is given.

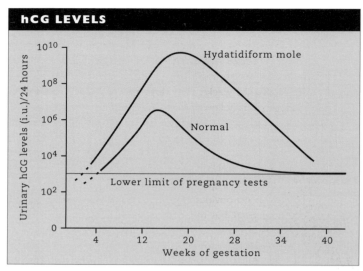

Fig. 3.6 Means of levels of hCG in women with normal pregnancies and hydatidiform moles.

A woman who has had a benign hydatidiform mole has a 1–4% chance of a repeat mole and so should have an early ultrasound scan in the next pregnancy.

LOCAL CAUSES OF BLEEDING

Cervicitis and vaginitis
- Occasional excessive infection (especially with *Candida*).
- Treat cause.

Cervical polyp
- Scanty bleeding. Can be seen with speculum.
- Leave alone in pregnancy and treat later if necessary.

Cervical erosion
- Spotting of blood only. Can be seen with speculum.
- Leave alone in pregnancy and treat later if necessary.

Varicosities of vagina
- Moderate bleeding in mid-trimester.
- Treat with pressure if close to vulva.
- Only ligate surgically in pregnancy if absolutely necessary.

Cancer of cervix

- Rare but important.
- Irregular bleeding and discharge. Confirm diagnosis by biopsy.
- If before 28 weeks, hysterotomy and immediate Wertheim hysterectomy followed by radiation.
- If after 28 weeks, may await 32–34 weeks then Caesarian Wertheim hysterectomy followed by radiation.

Urinary or anal bleeding may be reported as vaginal bleeding in error.

CAUSE NOT FOUND

This is a smaller group than that in late pregnancy bleeding. Many early bleeds of no obvious cause are labelled *threatened* miscarriage and so are diagnosed, but this is rarely proven. Hence *threatened* miscarriage is a loose diagnosis and includes many more women than are actually threatening to abort their fetus.

Genital tract bleeding in late pregnancy

Antepartum haemorrhage is defined as bleeding from the genital tract after the 24th week of pregnancy and before the onset of labour.

Incidence
5% of all pregnancies.

Causes

Maternal
- Placenta praevia: 30%.
- Abruptio placentae: 35%.
- Local cause in the vagina and cervix: 5%.
- Blood dyscrasias: <1%.
- Cause never found: 30%.

Fetal
Vasa praevia: <1%.

PLACENTA PRAEVIA

A placenta which encroaches on the lower segment of the uterus. The lower segment can be defined as that part of the uterine wall which:
- Does not contract in labour but is stretched in response to contractions.

- Used to be the isthmus before pregnancy.
- Underlies the loose fold of peritoneum that reflects from the bladder.
- Is covered by a full bladder anteriorly.
- Is within 8 cm of the internal cervical os at term.

Classification

Box 3.1 shows the classical, contemporary and ultrasound classifications. Figure 3.7 shows the stages of severity of a placenta praevia.

Aetiology

Placenta praevia follows the low implantation of the embryo. Associated factors are:

1 Multiparity.

2 Multiple pregnancy.

3 Embryos are more likely to implant on a lower segment scar from previous CS.

Presentation

- Nowadays most low-lying placentae or placentae praeviae are diagnosed by ultrasound.
- Recurrent painless bright red vaginal bleeding.
- A persistent malpresentation or high head in late pregnancy.

DEGREES OF PLACENTA PRAEVIA	
I	The placenta encroaches on the lower segment but does not reach the internal os
II	The placenta reaches the internal os of the cervix but does not cover it
III	The placenta covers the internal os before dilatation but not when dilated
IV	The placenta completely covers the internal os of the cervix even when dilated

Classical	Contemporary	Ultrasound
Type I	Marginal	Minor
Type II	Lateral	
Type III	Central	Major
Type IV		

Box 3.1 The classification of degrees of severity of a placenta praevia.

PLACENTA PRAEVIA

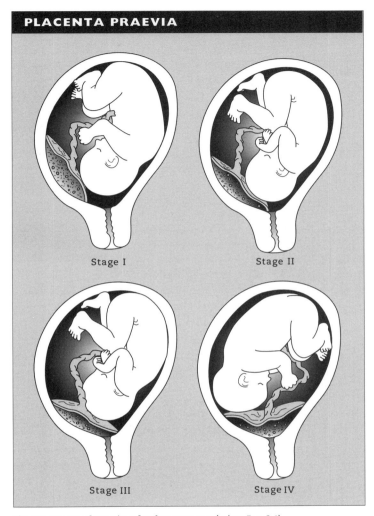

Stage I

Stage II

Stage III

Stage IV

Fig. 3.7 Stages of severity of a placenta praevia (see Box 3.1).

Ultrasound diagnosis

An ultrasound scan will show the position of the placenta clearly within the uterus (Fig. 3.8). If the placenta lies in the anterior part of the uterus and reaches into the area covered by the bladder, it is known as a low-lying placenta (before 24 weeks) and placenta praevia after 24 weeks.

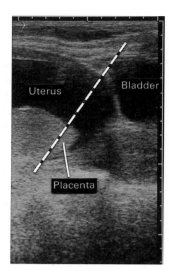

Fig. 3.8 Ultrasound scan showing posterior placenta praevia at 32 weeks' gestation. Dotted line is the junction of the upper and lower segments of the uterus.

Management

Asymptomatic low-lying placenta
- About 5% of pregnant women will have a low-lying placenta when scanned at 16–20 weeks' gestation.
- The incidence of placenta praevia at delivery is about 0.5%, therefore 9 out of 10 women convert.
- All women with a low-lying placenta diagnosed in early pregnancy should be rescanned at 34 weeks' gestation.
- There is no need to restrict work activities or sexual intercourse in women with a low-lying placenta on ultrasound only unless they bleed.
- If the placenta praevia is still present at 34 weeks' gestation and is of a minor degree, the woman should be rescanned on a fortnightly basis but need not be admitted to hospital unless bleeding occurs.
- There is, currently, no agreement amongst obstetricians whether women with a major degree of placenta praevia which is asymptomatic should be admitted but it seems a wise precaution.

Placenta praevia with bleeding
- Admit to hospital.
- Insert a broad-bore i.v. cannula and start an infusion of normal saline.
- Take blood for crossmatching and Hb estimation.

- *Avoid all digital vaginal examinations.* A gentle bivalve speculum examination may be performed later on women who are bleeding to determine if blood is coming through the cervical os, especially if a placenta praevia has been suspected but not diagnosed definitely.
- Perform ultrasound as soon as possible because this is more precise.
- All women who have bled during pregnancy with a placenta praevia should remain in hospital until delivery.
- Crossmatched blood should be kept permanently available.
- Placental position and fetal growth should be monitored by fortnightly ultrasound scans.
- At 36–37 weeks' presentation, a final ultrasound should be performed and acted upon:

  (a) Major degrees of placenta praevia should lead to a Caesarean section between 37 and 38 weeks' gestation by an experienced obstetrician.

  (b) If the presenting part is below the lower edge of the placenta, i.e. minor degrees of placenta praevia (I and II anterior), then it is safe to wait until labour and these women can be expected to deliver vaginally.

  With modern ultrasound there is little place for examination under anaesthetic.

Prognosis

Maternal
Death from placenta praevia in the developed world is now extremely rare. If women are in hospital Caesarean section should be undertaken to prevent death from excessive bleeding. The major cause of death in women with placenta praevia now is postpartum haemorrhage (PPH). PPH is common because the lower segment does not contract and retract as in the upper segment, and therefore maternal vessels of the placental bed may continue to bleed after delivery.

Fetal
Bleeding from placenta praevia is maternal in origin. The risk to the fetus is therefore entirely dependent upon the gestation at which it becomes necessary to deliver the baby.

PLACENTAL ABRUPTION

This is bleeding from the placental bed of a normally sited placenta. It may occur as an antepartum or an intrapartum event.

Classification

Major
This is clinically obvious and may result in the death of the fetus. It is also life-threatening to the mother and usually involves separation of more than one-third of the placenta.

Minor
Premature separation of small areas of the placenta may result in placental infarcts which can sometimes be seen on ultrasound. Several small abruptions may precede a large abruption. Much of the bleeding that occurs from an abruption is not discharged through the vagina and is known as concealed haemorrhage. Bleeding which is clinically obvious is revealed haemorrhage. Most are obviously mixed.

Aetiology
The causes of abruption are not known but the following factors are associated:
- Proteinuric hypertension.
- Multiparity. Fourth pregnancies carry a four times risk over first pregnancies.
- Trauma. External cephalic version and seat belt injuries.
- Overstretched uterus. Abruption usually occurs in this situation at the time that the membranes rupture.
- Previous placental abruption. This increases the risk by two to three times.
- Raised maternal serum α-fetoprotein (6% risk).

Presentation

Major
Women present with abdominal pain and varying degrees of shock. The blood loss that is visible (revealed haemorrhage) is often out of step with the degree of shock.
   On examination:
1 The uterus is woody hard; due to a tonic contraction.
2 The fetal parts cannot be felt.
3 The fetus may be dead.

Minor
Minor abruptions are often not diagnosed until after delivery. They may present with:

- Mild abdominal pain associated with threatened preterm labour.
- Unexplained APH.
- Tenderness over one area of the uterus only.

Complications

Severe abruption may result in:
- Shock from blood loss due to a large retroplacental clot, often concealed.
- A consumptive coagulopathy.
- Oliguria or anuria due to hypovolaemia.

Minor degrees of placental abruption may result in impaired fetal growth.

Management

Major placental abruption is a life-threatening condition for both the mother and the baby.

If the fetus is still alive, then respond as follows:

1 Insert two large-bore i.v. cannulae and infusion of normal saline.

2 Send 20 ml blood for crossmatch of 4 units, Hb and coagulation studies.

3 Perform an immediate Caesarean section if necessary to save the baby's life.

4 Ensure adequate fluid replacement following the Caesarean section.

5 Leave an indwelling urinary catheter into monitor urinary output.

If the fetus is dead, then the woman should be allowed to deliver vaginally. This usually happens rapidly (within 4–6 hours) as the abruption stimulates labour. If not in labour, rupture of membranes usually leads to a swift delivery. The relevant points of the management of labour are:

1 Insert two large-bore cannulae and start a saline infusion.

2 Send 20 ml blood for crossmatch of 4 units, Hb and coagulation studies.

3 Epidural analgesia is contra-indicated because of the risk of coagulopathy.

4 If a coagulopathy has developed or the woman starts to bleed, she should be managed in the following manner:

It should be done in conjunction with a consultant haematologist. Even if the coagulation studies are not available, coagulation failure usually becomes apparent if blood taken for blood tests has not clotted. If this occurs, then the following management is advised:

(a) Give 4 units of fresh frozen plasma.

(b) Ask the blood bank to get platelets of 6 units ready.

(c) Give platelets, cryoprecipitate or fibrinogen as advised by the consultant haematologist.

The consumptive coagulopathy begins to improve immediately after the uterus has been evacuated of its contents. Even marked abnormalities of the coagulation tests resolve within 4–6 hours of delivery of the placenta.

LOCAL CAUSES

These are discussed in the section on vaginal bleeding in early pregnancies (p. 82).

BLOOD DYSCRASIAS

These are extremely rare. Bleeding may be seen in the following conditions.

- Von Willebrand's disease.
- Leukaemia.
- Hodgkin's disease.
- Idiopathic thrombocytopenia.

Management

These conditions are usually known before pregnancy and are best managed in conjunction with a consultant haematologist or oncologist.

CAUSE NOT FOUND

Although the cause can often not be determined at the time that the bleeding occurs, careful pathological examination of the placenta will often reveal one of the following:

1 Rupture of the marginal sinus; this is a large vein that runs round the edge of the placenta and usually produces a single episode of painless bleeding, mimicking placenta praevia.

2 Placenta circumvallata. This is an unusual condition where the membranes insert some little distance along the placental surface. The area of the placenta not covered by the membranes then separates from the uterus and causes small episodes of painless recurrent vaginal bleeding mimicking placenta praevia. This is one of the few placental conditions that is known to impair fetal growth and is the reason why all women with an unexplained APH should have serial ultrasound examinations to monitor fetal growth.

3 The loss of the cervical mucous plug.

The complication rates from this group are small, especially if the fetus is growing normally. Many obstetricians however will induce, at term, women who have had an undiagnosed APH.

FETAL BLEEDING

This occurs from rupture of vasa praevia when there is a velamentous insertion of cord vessels and these cross the cervical os.

Diagnosis

This condition usually presents with scanty bleeding at the time of membrane rupture. It may be associated with alterations in the fetal heart rate producing a sinusoidal pattern (Fig. 3.9).

Confirmation

If there is time, the blood lost can be checked for fetal Hb by its resistance to alkalinization. Alternatively the condition may be suspected when an ultrasound examination reveals the presence of a succenturiate lobe on the opposite side of the internal os to the placenta.

Treatment

Deliver the fetus as soon as possible and prepare to transfuse.

Polyhydramnios

Best definition: an excess of amniotic fluid detected clinically. The range of

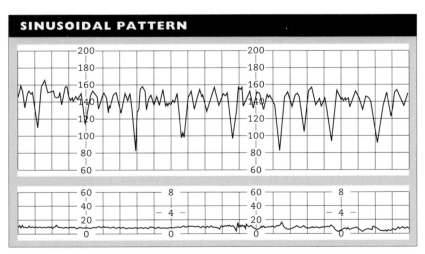

Fig. 3.9 CTG demonstrating a marked sinusoidal pattern together with probably early decelerations. The relationship of the decelerations to the contractions cannot be stated as the contractions have not registered.

normal volumes of fluid present is wide and varies with the duration of pregnancy. *Average* values for amniotic fluid are:

    12 weeks: 50 ml;
    24 weeks: 500 ml;
    36 weeks: 1000 ml;

but the normal range at term in a singleton pregnancy is large — 500–1500 ml.

Diagnosis

This is either clinical or a simple ultrasound. Other methods of measuring amniotic fluid *in situ* are too complex for routine use and often unreliable.

History
- Tenseness of abdomen.
- Unable to lie comfortably in any position.
- Dyspnoea, indigestion, piles and varicose veins.

Examination
- Girth of abdomen is increased.
- Very tense, cystic uterus bigger than maturity (like a balloon filled with water).
- Difficult to feel any fetal parts and impossible to grasp them.

Investigations
Ultrasound. The volume of fluid is represented by the longest column of free fluid from fetal surface to the internal uterine wall. In polyhydramnios the column is >8 cm.

Differential diagnosis
- Twins: laxer feel to uterus and many fetal parts felt.
- Ovarian cyst: uterus displaced to one side in later pregnancy.
- Full bladder: associated with uterus trapped in pelvis early in pregnancy.
- Hydatidiform mole: in earlier pregnancy only.
    All are resolved by ultrasound examination.

Associations

Maternal
- Diabetes.

Fetal
- Congenital abnormality; anencephaly; meningomyelocoele; bowel atresia.
- Twins (particularly monovular).

Clinical course

Acute
- Painful with tense uterus and oedematous abdominal wall.
- Primiparous.
- Pre-eclampsia.
- Often early (22–32 weeks' gestation).

Chronic
- Slower onset.
- Uncomfortable rather than painful.
- Last weeks of pregnancy.

Management

Acute
1 Bed rest.
2 Ultrasound to rule out twins or abnormality.
3 Release fluid from uterus.
   - If *fetus normal*: through abdominal wall with narrow-bore needle. Drain fluid off slowly until the woman is comfortable (500–1000 ml over 4–8 hours).
   - If *fetus abnormal* and viable — consider induction. If not viable — paracentesis.

Chronic
1 Bed rest.
2 Ultrasound to rule out twins and fetal abnormality.
3 Sedation if very painful.
4 Treat underlying maternal condition.
5 If fetus normal, induce labour when indicated by fetal state *not* because of the polyhydramnios.
6 Watch for uterine dysfunction and PPH in labour.

Oligohydramnios

A lack of amniotic fluid, a much rarer condition.

Diagnosis
- Uterus is small for dates (early).
- Uterus feels full of fetus (later).
- Ultrasound shows small (<2 cm) columns.

Fetal associations
- Adhesions from fetal skin to amnion.
- Renal agenesis.
- IUGR.

Clinical course
- Labour often preterm.
- High fetal death rate.
- High rate of fetal abnormalities (e.g. dislocated hips and talipes).

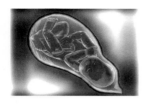

Diseases in Pregnancy

Urinary tract infection in pregnancy

During pregnancy the ureters are dilated and kinked because of:
- Increased progesterone levels which relax the smooth muscle.
- Mild obstruction of the lower ureters in late pregnancy.

This encourages:
- Stasis of urine.
- Reflux of infected urine to the kidney evoking pyelonephritis.

ASYMPTOMATIC BACTERIURIA

The presence of more than 10^5 bacteria/ml of urine in the absence of symptoms.

Incidence
About 5% of pregnant women — increases with parity and age.

Significance
Asymptomatic bacteriuria is associated with a risk of:
- Acute pyelonephritis in pregnancy (30%).
- Structural abnormalities in the urinary tract (3–5%).

Screening
In early pregnancy, all women should have urine tested for either:
- The presence of white cells.
- Cultured for bacteria.

Treatment
The most common organisms grown are:

- *Escherichia coli.*
- *Proteus mirabilis.*

These are usually sensitive to amoxycillin, trimethoprim or nitrofurantoin. A 14-day course of an antibiotic to which the organism is sensitive should be prescribed. This will result in a cure in more than 85% of women but the urine should be recultured 1 week after treatment.

A renal ultrasound and an i.v. urogram should be performed 3 months after delivery to exclude a structural urinary tract abnormality.

SYMPTOMATIC INFECTIONS

Incidence
1–2%; commoner in primigravidae.

Symptoms
- Dysuria (due to urethritis).
- Increased frequency (due to trigonitis).
- Backache, loin pains, night sweats and rigors (due to pyelonephritis).
- Headache, vomiting and muscle aches (due to pyrexia).

Examination
- The woman is usually pyrexial if the infection has involved the kidneys. In many cases this may be at levels of up to 40.5°C.
- If the woman has pyelonephritis she will be tender in the renal angles.

Investigation
A mid-stream specimen of urine (MSU) should be sent for:
- Microscopy for white cells.
- Culture to determine the organism responsible.
- Sensitivity of organisms to antibiotics.

Management
All women who have renal angle tenderness or a pyrexia must be admitted to hospital because of the threat of preterm labour.

Management consists of:

1   Bed rest.

2   Ample fluid intake, at least 3 litres a day; if nauseated, give i.v.

3   Start a broad-spectrum i.v. antibiotic such as amoxycillin; may change when an organism's antibiotic sensitivities are known.

4   If the woman has pyelonephritis, do a renal ultrasound when she has recovered from the infection.

5   Keep her in hospital until the renal angle tenderness has disappeared.

6   The antibiotics can be given orally once temperature is normal. A complete 7-day course at least should be given. The urine should be recultured 2 days after the last dose of antibiotic has been given.

CHRONIC RENAL DISEASE

Renal changes in normal pregnancy
- Renal blood flow increases.
- Glomerular filtration rate (GFR) increases.
- Plasma concentrations of urea and creatinine fall in normal pregnancy.
- There is an increase in total body water that exceeds the increase in total body sodium, resulting in a decrease in plasma osmolality.
- There is a 25% fall in serum uric acid concentrations during the first two trimesters but this returns to pre-pregnant levels by the third trimester.

Prognosis
The prognosis for the pregnancy depends upon:
1   Whether the woman was hypertensive before pregnancy.
2   Whether the woman had proteinuria before pregnancy started.
3   The type of renal disease.
   Pregnancy probably has no long-term adverse effects on renal disease.

Fetal prognosis
- Normotensive women with chronic renal disease have a × 2–3 greater risk of developing PIH (pre-eclampsia). In the absence of PIH perinatal mortality is not increased. If PIH develops, the risk of fetal death is directly related to the gestation of delivery.
- Women with more severe renal disease have a high incidence of both PIH and impaired fetal growth. Among women with pre-existing hypertension and proteinuria, the perinatal mortality rates approach 30%. Cause of death is from preterm delivery and complications associated with SGA.

Women on haemodialysis
- Women on regular haemodialysis are not infertile and many ovulate regularly.
- There is a high incidence of preterm delivery.
- Preterm contractions commonly start during or immediately after dialysis.
- Women on dialysis should have appropriate contraceptive advice and ideally should postpone pregnancy until after transplantation.

Pregnancy following renal transplantation

- Menstruation normally reappears in women with chronic renal disease within 6 months of a successful transplant. This restores fertility to normal. If pregnancy is not sought, ensure contraception.
- There is no evidence that pregnancy increases the incidence of renal rejection.
- Proteinuric hypertension occurs $\times$ 3–4 more frequently after transplantation.
- Up to 40% of fetuses will be delivered preterm; survival depends upon the gestational age at delivery.
- There is little evidence that immunosuppressant drugs or steroids increase the risk of congenital abnormalities.

Acute renal failure in pregnancy

This may be:

1 Tubular necrosis: this is largely recoverable.

2 Cortical necrosis: this is usually irrecoverable and these patients go on to need long-term dialysis or transplantation.

Presentation

1 Oliguria: <500 ml/day (20 ml/hour), the minimum volume to remove catabolites.

2 Anuria: the absence of urine.

Aetiology in obstetrics

1 *Hypovolaemia.*
  - Severe pre-eclampsia.
  - Miscarriage.
  - Placental abruption.
  - PPH.
  - Hyperemesis gravidarum.

2 *Gram-negative shock.* This may result from:
  - Septic miscarriage.
  - Pyelonephritis.
  - Chorioamnionitis.
  - Puerperal infections.

The usual organism is *E. coli*; but it may be *Clostridium*.

3 *Nephrotoxins.* In modern obstetric practice these are rare. Illegal abortions may result in infection followed by haemolysis and renal failure.

4 *Acute renal failure* associated with acute fatty liver of pregnancy. Rare; usually fatal.

5 *Vomiting* in late pregnancy associated with jaundice. The disease occurs in many systems and renal failure, pancreatitis and colitis may occur.

Management

Three consecutive phases:

1 *Oliguria*: lasts from a few days to a few weeks. Complete anuria is rare in acute tubular necrosis and usually suggests acute cortical necrosis or obstruction.

2 *Polyuria*: markedly increased urine production that may last up to 2 weeks. The urine is dilute and metabolic waste products are poorly eliminated. Plasma urea and creatinine may continue to rise for several days following the increase in urinary output. Profound fluid and electrolyte losses can occur in this phase.

3 *Recovery*: urinary volumes decrease towards normal and renal function improves.

General management:
- Determine the cause.
- Insert a urinary catheter and maintain accurate fluid balance charts.
- Insert a central venous pressure line and measure the pressure.

In pregnancy, central venous pressure should range from $+4$ to $+10\,cmH_2O$. If this is low it suggests the cause of the renal failure is due to hypovolaemia and therefore the volume should be restored with up to 2 litres of normal saline followed by a plasma expander. Response of over 30 ml of urine in 1 hour should be seen within 1 hour of the fluid load.

- Send baseline investigations including urea and electrolytes, liver function tests, serum amylase, plasma proteins, coagulation studies and if required perform an arterial blood sample for acid–base balance.
- If the patient is not hypovolaemic or does not respond to the fluid load, then the alternatives are as follows:

    (a) Conservative management. Give the patient fluid output plus 500 ml/day. Monitor electrolytes and start dialysis if and when the patient is uraemic or hypercataebolic.

    (b) Intensive management using vasodilators. This requires the insertion of a pulmonary artery catheter and the monitoring of cardiac output. Vasodilators are given and the patient is fluid-loaded.

- Involve intensive care physicians or the renal physician at an early stage.

Anaemia

Anaemia can follow:

1 Lack of production of blood: haemopoietic.

2 Increased breakdown of blood: haemolytic.

3 Blood loss: haemorrhagic.

In pregnancy, most anaemia is haemopoietic when it may be due to lack of:

1 Iron: iron deficiency anaemia.

2 Folic acid: megaloblastic anaemia.

3 Protein: iron deficiency anaemia.

Normal levels of haematological indices are shown in Box 4.1.

IRON DEFICIENCY ANAEMIA

Aetiology

Poor intake
- Diet deficient in iron-containing foods.

Poor absorption
- Vomiting in pregnancy affects absorption.
- Increased pH of gastric juice.
- Ferric ions in gut instead of ferrous.
- Lack of vitamin C.

Increased utilization
Demands of pregnancy. Total body iron measures about 3500 mg. Includes:
- Fetus and uterus: 500 mg.
- Increased maternal blood volume: 500 mg.

HAEMATOLOGICAL VALUES IN PREGNANCY

Blood	Range
Total blood volume (ml)	4000–6000
Red cell volume (ml)	1500–1800
Red cell count (10^{12}/l)	4–5
White cell count (10^9/l)	8–18
Haemoglobin (g/dl)	10.5–13.5
Erythrocyte sedimentation rate (mm in the first hour)	10–60
Mean corpuscular volume (fl)	80–95
Mean corpuscular haemoglobin (μg)	32–36
Serum iron (μmol/l)	11–25
Serum ferritin (μg/l)	10–200
Serum folate (μg/l)	6–9
Total iron-binding capacity (μmol/l)	40–70

Box 4.1 Normal haematological values in pregnancy.

More if:
- Multiple pregnancies.
- Too many pregnancies.
- Pregnancies close together.

Diagnosis
- Rarely made clinically unless woman is severely affected.
- May have tiredness and oedema.
- May show pallor of conjunctivae.
- Hb estimates must be done on all pregnant women at booking, and twice later in pregnancy, such as at 28 and 34 weeks.
- If level below 10 g/dl, diagnose anaemia and look for cause.

Haematology (Box 4.2)
Iron deficiency anaemia may show:
- Changed red blood cells:
    (a) Microcytic: smaller.
    (b) Anisocytic: variations in size.
    (c) Poikilocytic: variations in shape.
- Hb level low.
- Serum iron (below 70 µg/dl).
- Reticulocytes: increase indicates response of bone marrow to stimulus of treatment.

IRON DEFICIENCY ANAEMIA

Blood film
Red cells
   Normal size or microcytic
   Hypochromic
   Anisocytosis
   Poikilocytosis

Haematological values
Haemoglobin ↓
Mean corpuscular volume ↓
Mean corpuscular haemoglobin ↓
Mean corpuscular haemoglobin C ↓
Serum iron ↓
Serum ferritin ↓

Box 4.2 Indices of iron deficiency anaemia.

Treatment

Preventive

Regular iron-bearing foods in diet (Box 4.3). If needed, iron tablet supplements. Daily requirements are 100 mg elemental iron with 300 μg folic acid.

* See she gets them — give them to her at the clinics.
* See she takes them — ask repeatedly.
* See they are effective — check Hb levels.

Curative

Depends on:

1   Degree of anaemia.
2   Duration of pregnancy.
3   Cause for iron deficiency:
   * Mild anaemia: Hb below 10 g/dl.
   * Severe anaemia: Hb below 8 g/dl.
   Mild:

1   Check that the woman is being given and is taking oral iron.
2   If so, increase oral iron or try another preparation.
3   If not, use another preparation.
4   If she cannot swallow tablets, use liquid preparation.
5   If change of oral therapy does not improve, use i.m. or i.v. preparation.
6   Give total dose i.v. as a transfusion in 1000 ml of saline. Alternatively, iron dextran 250 mg is associated with rise of Hb of about 1 g/dl. Give on alternate days, i.m. for six doses with small test dose first to check anaphylaxis.

   Severe and early:

IRON-RICH FOODS

Animal
Red meat—iron in haemoglobin and myoglobin
White meat ⎫
Fish   ⎭ iron in the myoglobin

Plant
Lentils
Dark-green leaf vegetables ⎫ moderate amount of iron only (rich in
Beans of all sorts   ⎭ folates)

Box 4.3 The iron-rich foods.

1   Admit to hospital and check that anaemia is solely iron deficient:
- Blood film.
- Serum iron.
- Total iron-binding capacity.
- Serum ferritin.
- Serum folate.

2   Treat with i.m. or i.v. therapy.

3   Check that protein and vitamin intake is adequate.

4   Check that improvement is maintained for rest of pregnancy.

Severe and late:

1   If after 36 weeks, too late to rely on haemopoiesis to provide red cells in time to cover labour. Therefore transfuse with packed red cell blood.

2   If Hb below 4 g/dl consider exchange transfusion.

3   Build up iron stores for puerperium by i.m. therapy.

FOLIC ACID DEFICIENCY ANAEMIA

Aetiology

Folic acid required for building DNA in all tissues. Hence demands are maximal when fetal tissue being made.

1   Poor intake:
- Diet deficient in folates.
- Vomiting in pregnancy.

2   Increased utilization:
- Demands of pregnancy.
- Rapid growth of fetal, placental and uterine tissues.
- Worse if:
    - (a) Multiple pregnancy.
    - (b) Grand multiparity.
    - (c) Fetal haemolysis (in Rh effect).
    - (d) Infection.

Commoner in underdeveloped countries and combined with other forms of malnutrition.

Diagnosis

Sometimes made clinically.
- May be tired, breathless, oedematous.
- May have other signs of malnutrition.

Haematology

See Box 4.4.

MEGALOBLASTIC ANAEMIA

Blood film
Red cells
    Normal size or macrocytic
    Normochromic
    Anisocytosis
    Poikilocytosis
    Sometimes nuclear cells
White cells
    Leucopenia
    Sometimes hypersegmentation
Platelets
    Sometimes thrombocytopenia

Haematological values
Haemoglobin ↓
Mean corpuscular volume ↑ or =
Mean corpuscular haemoglobin C ↑
Serum iron ↑
Serum folate ↓

Marrow
Megaloblasts ↑

Box 4.4 Indices of megaloblastic anaemia.

Treatment

Preventive
Folic acid supplements in last 20 weeks of pregnancy (300 μg/day).

Theoretical risk of masking pernicious anaemia (PA) and its uncommon accompanying subacute combined degeneration (SCD) of the spinal cord. In practice, PA is very rare in those under 35 years and SCD almost unknown in the pregnancy age group.

Curative
• Mild or moderate anaemia — folic acid 5–10 mg/day orally only.
• Severe anaemia — folic acid 5–10 mg/day i.m.:
    (a) oral iron
    (b) blood transfusion } both should be given with care.

HAEMOLYTIC ANAEMIA

These can all be diagnosed before pregnancy at pre-pregnancy consultation.

Thalassaemia

Aetiology
Defective formation of Hb side chains. May be α or β which can either be:
- Homozygous — thalassaemia major: usually fatal and does not concern obstetricians.
- Heterozygous — thalassaemia minor: commonest thalassaemia.

β-thalassaemia minor is the more serious especially if combined with any other abnormal Hb such as S or C.

Diagnosis
- Classically women from the Mediterranean countries but now widespread in the Middle and Far East. The woman usually knows about this and will mention it in the history.
- Can be picked up from electrophoresis of blood.
- Occasionally a mild anaemia.
- Splenomegaly.
- Jaundice.
- Pain from bone infarcts (later in life — ulcers of legs).

Haematology
- Increased red blood cell fragility.
- Hb level low.
- Serum iron raised.

Treatment
1 No use giving iron alone (iron stores high) but folate helpful.
2 Cover haemolytic crisis with transfusions carefully.
3 Prevent stress if possible (e.g. hypoxia).
4 Treat infections early.
5 Beware coexistent:
   - Malaria.
   - Glucose-6-phosphate dehydrogenase deficiency.
   - Other abnormal Hb.
6 Deliver between crises.

Haemoglobinopathies

Aetiology
- Defective genes alter side chains in Hb.
- Red blood cells containing such Hb break down more easily than normal.

- Abnormal Hb:
  (a) HbS (commonest): Middle East, Africa, USA and southern Europe.
  (b) HbC: Ghana.
  (c) HbE: South East Asia.
  (d) HbD: Punjab.

Diagnosis

- Crises or infarcts:
  (a) Chest pain.
  (b) Sudden head or abdominal pain.
- Bone marrow exhaustion.

Haematology

- Low Hb.
- Sickling and target cells on blood film (Box 4.5).
- Electrophoresis shows abnormal Hb patterns.
- C crystals.

Treatment

1 Detect early.
2 Folic acid prophylactically 1–2 mg/day.
3 Transfused with packed red blood cells with a diuretic at the same time.
4 Prevent:

SICKLE CELL ANAEMIA

Blood film
Red cells
    Polychromatophilia
    Sickle cells
    Anisocytosis
    Poikilocytosis
    ? Howell–Jolly bodies
White cells
    Leucocytosis
Platelets
    Thrombocytosis

Check
Haemoglobin electrophoresis

Box 4.5 Indices of sickle cell anaemia.

- Hypoxia.
- Dehydration.
- Trauma.
- A splenectomy for some.

5 If crisis:
- Check Hb every 4 hours.
- Heparinize.
- Consider exchange transfusion.
- If blood pressure rises rapidly, deliver.

HAEMORRHAGIC ANAEMIA
Rare in temperate climates:
- Recurrent chronic gastrointestinal bleeding (peptic ulcer, piles).

Commoner in tropics:
- Recurrent chronic bleeding (e.g. tapeworms, hookworms).

Treatment
- Treat cause
- Correct anaemia — as above.

Heart disease

Frequency and severity of heart disease in pregnancy are diminishing in this country because:
- Most heart disease in this age group is rheumatic in origin.
- Rheumatic fever is much rarer in childhood with better housing and nutrition.
- Rheumatic fever is more effectively treated in childhood by chemotherapy.

Aetiology
- Rheumatic 80%: mitral valve affected 85%, aortic valve 10%, both 5%.
- Congenital 15%: septal defects and reversed shunts.
- All the rest 5%: ischaemic, thyrotoxic, syphilitic.

Pathophysiology
Pregnancy is a hyperkinetic state and is an extra load on the heart. If the heart is damaged, avoid other loads.
- Anaemia — dilute blood is inefficient.
- Pre-eclampsia — harder work if hypertension or oedema present.
- Arrhythmia — fibrillation is inefficient at delivering blood.
- Flare-up of rheumatic fever — not common but watch for and treat.

• Acute bacterial endocarditis risk increased because of irregular endothelium over heart valves; hence cover surgery and dentistry with antibiotics.

Cardiac complications in pregnancy

1 With mitral stenosis:
• Pulmonary oedema: especially if tight valve and small heart. This is the commonest and often occurs in late pregnancy or immediately postpartum.
• Right-sided congestive failure: especially in women who have had congestive cardiac failure (CCF) before. Rare to start *de novo* in pregnancy.

2 With aortic stenosis:
• Left-sided congestive failure. Rare to start *de novo*, in pregnancy.

3 Eisenmenger's syndrome.
• If right-to-left shunt or bidirectional one, high risk of pulmonary hypertension.

4 Fallot's tetralogy.
• Lower resistance at pulmonary valve and right ventricular out-flow tract — less risk of failure. If right-to-left shunt — high risk of failure.

5 Coarctation of aorta.
• Common in the pregnancy age group. Risks of rupture in late pregnancy or labour. Often repaired before; if well healed, no increased dangers.

Management

In pregnancy
1 Diagnose early.
• History.
• Examination.

2 Assess severity early: ideally cardiologist and obstetrician to see woman together, at antenatal clinic.
• Investigations.
• ECG.
• Chest X-ray.
• Echocardiography.
• Maybe:
   (a) Catheter studies (pressure and blood gases).
   (b) 24-hour ECG.
• Factors:
   (a) Age.

(b) Severity of lesion.

(c) Functional decompensation.

3 Book for hospital delivery and be prepared for bed rest in hospital.

4 Extra rest at home.

5 Continue anticoagulation if patient already on it. Consider subcutaneous heparin rather than oral anticoagulants unless plastic valve prosthesis. For these continue on warfarin.

6 Senior cardiologist, anaesthetist and obstetrician make labour plan and write it on hospital records. See that senior staff of each discipline are available to cover labour.

In labour

1 Reduce extra work — good analgesia; probably epidural unless anticoagulated.

2 Nurse head up: tilt bed or pillows.

3 Antibiotics especially if a congenital heart lesion.

4 Short second stage; maybe forceps or vacuum extraction.

5 Give Syntometrine if high risk of PPH; otherwise not.

6 Manage pulmonary oedema if it occurs.

- Tilt head up 35°.
- O_2.
- Aminophylline 0.5 g, i.v.
- Morphine 15 mg.
- Digitalis if arrhythmia or tachycardia.
- Diuretics — frusemide.

In puerperium

1 Rest:

- Keep in hospital longer.
- Check home conditions adequate — few stairs if possible.

2 Physiotherapy to legs and gentle exercises.

3 Breast feeding allowed unless cardiac condition deteriorated in pregnancy. It can be hard work, for only one person can do it and it means getting up at night.

Prognosis

Maternal

1 Mortality: increased risk of death — 9% of all maternal deaths in UK are associated with heart disease.

2 Morbidity: increased risk of deterioration of heart condition. Used to be inevitable. This is not so if proper care is taken.

Fetal
Little increased risk if mother kept healthy. Watch for fetal risks from anti-coagulation if relevant.

Respiratory diseases

PULMONARY TUBERCULOSIS

Incidence
Less than 1:1000 in UK; rare in endogenous population, higher in immigrants (e.g. Indian born have a $\times$ 6–10 greater prevalence than among British born).

Presentation
- History of disease and treatments often known to woman.
- Pick up on routine chest X-ray.
- Rarely clinically diagnosed from physical signs.

Management
1   Notify any new cases to District Public Health Specialist.
2   Continue any antituberculous drugs already started in combination:
   - Streptomycin.*
   - INAH (isonicotinic hydrazide).
   - Ethambutol.
   - Rifampicin.*
*Beware potential teratogenic effect in first trimester.
3   Bed rest.
4   Surgery if needed in mid-pregnancy, avoiding first 14 and last 10 weeks.
5   Follow up the family.

Labour
Delivery by most expeditious route (fetus may be large).

Mother
1   Allow breast feeding if no positive sputum bacteriology within 1 year and no chest X-ray signs of recent activity.
2   Continue all drug treatments.
3   Suppress lactation if baby has to be separated.
4   Rest in hospital longer.
5   Check community back-up services to give least effort to mother.

6 Arrange for follow-up at chest clinic in case of tuberculosis flare-up.

Baby
1 If mother has had bacteria in sputum within 1 year, separate baby from mother at birth. The mother must be warned during pregnancy that this will happen. If properly explained, she will realize it is a wise move.
2 Give baby isoniazid-resistant BCG 0.05 mg at 7 days (unless premature). Await positive Mantoux before allowing baby back to mother (about 6 weeks).

ASTHMA

In pregnancy
Often emotional factors are involved so asthma may worsen if pregnancy is resented. Continue all treatments started before pregnancy. Be careful of new therapies, e.g. budesonide may be teratogenic to some species. Not known to be so in humans. Therefore use well-established drugs.
- Bronchial antispasmodics.
- Antibiotics.

  Most asthmatics do not deteriorate in pregnancy but may in puerperium. No obvious correlation with hormone changes.

In labour
1 Deliver so that mother's respiratory effort is minimal.
2 May require extra antispasmodics in labour.
3 If on steroids, hydrocortisone required to cover labour.
4 Baby may be small for dates if asthma control was poor.

Endocrine diseases

THYROID DISEASE
Pregnancy is a hyperdynamic state. Increased oestrogen levels cause enlargement of thyroid gland and an increased output of thyroid hormone. Since this is mostly in the form of protein-bound thyroxine, such patients are not hyperthyroid, for the active fraction is not increased.

Hyperthyroidism
- Difficult to diagnose for the first time in pregnancy.
- If established beforehand, continue treatment; usually carbimazole, but keep dose as low as possible.

- Consider thyroidectomy if disease is increasingly difficult to control. Operation is safe if mother properly prepared. Avoid radioactive-iodine testing because of fetal thyroid pick-up and retention. Maternal thyroid-stimulating IgG pass across placenta and may stimulate fetal thyroid, sometimes enough to cause neonatal thyrotoxicosis. This is unusual but can be predicted by testing maternal blood levels of IgG in late pregnancy.

Hypothyroidism
- Rarely get pregnant if not on therapy.
- If treated, continue treatment, and be prepared to increase dosage.

ADRENAL DISEASE
Normally there are increased cortisol levels in pregnancy because:
- Raised adrenal cortex secretion.
- Decreased metabolism of steroid.
  90% of circulating cortisol is bound to globulin and is inactive.

Hypoadrenalism (Addison's disease)
- Usually well balanced on replacement cortisone.
- Be prepared to increase dose particularly during vomiting or labour.
- Puerperal diuresis may deplete sodium.

Hyperadrenalism (Cushing's syndrome)
- Pregnancy rare since women with this syndrome usually do not ovulate.
- Metyrapone (aldosterone inhibitor) if high cortisol levels.
- Watch for hypertension.
- Preterm delivery common.
- Watch for androgenic effects on fetus.

PITUITARY DISEASE

Prolactinoma
- Women on long-term bromocriptine become pregnant on it.
- Oestrogen stimulation of pregnancy may cause enlargement of tumour; pressure on optic chiasma threatens vision.
- Check with CT scan. Prolactin levels raised but variable.
- A few tumours need treatment if they enlarge:
  (a) first bromocriptine;
  (b) then surgery.

Acromegaly

- Rarely become pregnant.
- Treat as prolactinoma.
- Baby often normal (growth hormone does not cross the placenta).

Hypopituitarism

- Mostly starts in puerperium after pituitary vein thrombosis following PPH.
- Study each pituitary function, separate and treat those deficient.
- If mother treated, baby does well.

DIABETES

Diabetes is a metabolic disease which results from an underproduction of insulin by the pancreas. This results in disturbances of carbohydrate, fat and protein metabolism and leads to sustained rise in blood glucose.

During pregnancy, diabetes may be one of the following types:

1 Pre-existing diabetes which is usually insulin-dependent.

2 Diabetes or an impaired glucose tolerance test discovered for the first time in pregnancy; gestational diabetes.

Glucose homeostasis in pregnancy

- In normal pregnancy, fasting glucose blood levels are maintained at 4–5 mmol/l.
- To maintain the glucose level, however, there is a doubling in the secretion of insulin from the end of the first to the third trimester of pregnancy. Pregnancy respresents a relatively insulin-resistant state.
- The insulin resistance is due to the placental secretion of oestrogen, progestogen and human placental lactogen together with a change in peripheral insulin receptors.
- Glucose crosses the placenta by facilitated diffusion so that the fetus has a glucose level of approximately 1 mmol/l less than its mother.
- The facilitated diffusion system is saturated at maternal levels of 11–12 mol/l. Therefore the fetus is probably never subject to levels of greater than 11 mmol/l.

Established diabetes mellitis

Occurs in 1–2% of the pregnant population.

Effects of pregnancy on the diabetes

- Insulin requirements increase during pregnancy and rapidly fall to pre-pregnancy levels after delivery.

- Pregnancy aggravates proliferative diabetic retinopathy. This may result in a vitreous haemorrhage and blindness. Previously proliferative retinopathy in early pregnancy was an indication for termination but now it can be dealt with by laser therapy. Ideally any retinopathy should be treated before pregnancy.
- Women with diabetic nephropathy are more likely to develop pre-eclampsia and to demonstrate temporary deteriorating renal function during pregnancy.
- There is a high incidence of IUGR and preterm delivery.
- There is no evidence that pregnancy has any adverse long-term effects on renal function.
- Diabetic neuropathy and vascular disease are rarely seen in women of reproductive age.

Effects of the diabetes on the pregnancy

- Poorly controlled diabetic women are sub-fertile; improving control increases their fertility.
- Increase in first trimester miscarriages.
- Increase in second trimester miscarriages, particularly those associated with death of the fetus.
- Increase in congenital abnormalities. This is increased by some $\times$ 3 to about 6%. The distribution of abnormalities is the same in diabetics as in the background population (50% neural tube defects, 30% cardiac abnormalities). Diabetics tend to show a predominance of multiple malformations and the unusual malformation of the caudal regression syndrome almost exclusively appears in diabetics.
- Increase in the incidence of pregnancy-induced hypertension.
- Increase in the incidence of preterm delivery.
- Increase in the incidence of polyhydramnios.
- Increased risk of sudden intrauterine death in the last 4 weeks of pregnancy. This appears to be confined to babies who are macrosomic.
- Increased incidence of macrosomic infants which may result in difficulties at delivery particularly shoulder dystocia.
- The overall increase in perinatal mortality is $\times$ 2–3 that of the total population but this can be reduced to background levels with good care.

Effects of diabetes on the infant

- Macrosomia: birth weight for gestational age exceeds the 90th centile.
- An increased risk of birth trauma, because of shoulder dystocia.
- An increased risk of asphyxia during delivery.

- An increased risk of respiratory distress syndrome (RDS) compared with babies of similar gestation.
- Hypoglycaemia. The fetal pancreas secretes high levels of insulin during pregnancy to cope with the passage of glucose from the mother. After delivery, the glucose source is removed, but the pancreas continues to secrete extra insulin resulting in hypoglycaemia.
- Hypercalcaemia.
- Hypothermia. Infants with diabetic mothers have large surface areas and so lose heat rapidly. Although they have more fat than the normal baby, this is yellow fat and is not the thermogenic brown fat.
- Hyperbilirubinaemia. Infants with diabetic mothers are plethoric due to polycythaemia and the excess red blood cells break down after delivery causing jaundice.

Management

There is increasing evidence that good control of diabetes around the time of conception, and the first weeks after, reduces the incidence of congenital abnormalities and of miscarriage. Good control throughout pregnancy reduces many of the complications but does not seem to affect the incidence of macrosomia (approximately 30%).

Pre-pregnancy care

- All insulin-dependent diabetics of reproductive age should take adequate contraceptive precautions until ready for pregnancy.
- Stress the need for pre-pregnancy counselling and planning:

    (a) If they are on oral hypoglycaemic agent they should be changed to insulin.

    (b) Twice-daily insulin regimens are the minimum acceptable for pregnancy. The best control of diabetes is achieved by giving a long-acting insulin at night and then by using a short-acting insulin to cover each meal throughout the day.
- Women should be taught to monitor their own blood sugar by BM Stix or Dextrostix. The monitoring should preferably be done by using an electronic glucose meter as well as the sticks.
- Blood sugar should be monitored first thing in the morning, 1 hour before each meal and 1 hour after the biggest meal of the day.
- The aim is to maintain the blood sugar between 4 and 9 mmol/l.
- HbA, level should be checked after 6 weeks on the above regimen and should be less than 8%.

Pregnancy management

This should ideally be done in a joint clinic in which women are seen by a

diabetic physician with an interest in obstetrics and an obstetrician with an interest in diabetes.
- The aim is to maintain normoglycaemia as described above, throughout the pregnancy. This may lead to an increase in the number of hypoglycaemic attacks but these are not harmful to the fetus.
- The fetal death rate with hyperglycaemic coma is as high as 25%.
- The woman should be seen fortnightly throughout her pregnancy.
- Management of pregnant diabetics can normally be achieved at home especially if a specialist diabetic nurse is available to give advice over the telephone or to visit the patient's home.
- At each antenatal visit the following should be checked:
    (a) The woman's diabetic record of home monitoring should be reviewed.
    (b) The blood pressure.
    (c) Symptoms suggestive of infection, particularly in the urinary tract.
    (d) Fetal growth by clinical means and by reviewing the ultrasound results.
- The insulin requirements will increase markedly during pregnancy. In the first trimester they are usually static but then increase rapidly until 34 weeks, when they may then stabilize. Women should be taught to change their own insulin dosage.

Ultrasound investigations
1 At 7 weeks' gestation to confirm fetal life and the number of fetuses.
2 At 16–20 weeks' gestation a detailed scan for structural abnormalities.
3 At 22–24 weeks' gestation to look specifically for cardiac abnormalities.
4 Insulin-dependent diabetes alone is not an indication to perform karyotyping.
5 Monthly fetal growth and amniotic fluid volume monitored. Figure 4.1 demonstrates the pattern of growth that is observed in babies who are destined to be macrosomic.

Delivery
- Induce labour usually between 38 and 41 weeks' gestation.
- Caesarean section should only be carried out on obstetric grounds.
- Control of diabetes during labour is achieved by i.v. insulin infusion together with i.v. glucose. The woman's blood glucose is checked every hour by means of BM Stix, and should be 4–10 mmol/l.
- She should be encouraged to have an epidural as pain and fear release catecholamines which are gluconeogenic.

FETAL MACROSOMIA

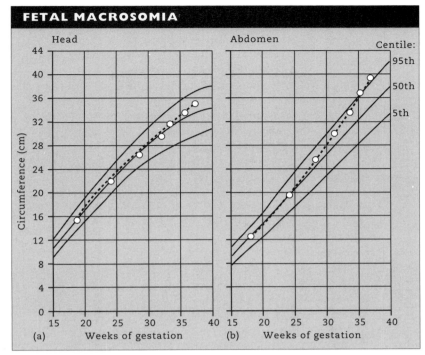

Fig 4.1 Ultrasound growth charts showing a case of fetal macrosomia.
(a) Head circumference. (b) Abdominal circumference.

- Labour should be accelerated with Syntocinon if readings are more than 2 hours to the right of the partogram (see Chapter 5).
- A senior obstetrician should be present at the delivery because of the risk of shoulder dystocia.
- The incidence of Caesarean section in insulin-dependent diabetics is × 2–3 higher than the normal population because:
  - (a) Failed induction.
  - (b) Fetal distress in early labour.
  - (c) Cephalopelvic disproportion.
  - (d) An abnormal lie.

Immediate care of the baby

A paediatrician should be present at the delivery of all babies of insulin-dependent diabetic mothers. The following features are important:
- Resuscitate the baby if required.

- Dry the baby and keep it warm.
- Perform a BM Stix estimation of glucose from a heel prick at: 30 minutes, 1 hour, 4 hours, 8 hours, 12 hours and 24 hours.
- To prevent hypoglycaemia feed the baby early with glucose solution.
- Treat low values of blood glucose (less than 1 mmol/l) with an i.v. infusion of glucose. Some babies are resistant and may need to be given i.m. glucagon.
- Carefully examine the baby for congenital abnormalities.
- Measure the serum bilirubin on the 2nd day as this is when the hyperbilirubinaemia usually starts.

Gestational diabetes

This is defined as the onset of diabetes or the appearance of abnormal glucose tolerance for the first time during pregnancy. A small proportion of these women will remain diabetic after delivery.

Gestational diabetes is not associated with congenital abnormalities. Main effects are:

- Development of polyhydramnios.
- Increase in the incidence of preterm labour.
- Production of macrosomia.

It can be screened for in the following ways:

1   Glucose tolerance test (GTT) on women at high-risk (Table 4.1).
2   Oral glucose load and a single blood sugar estimation 2 hours later.
3   Random blood sugar at 28 weeks' gestation related to the time of the last meal. Women who have high blood sugars are then given a glucose tolerance test.

The glucose tolerance test

This is a 75-g oral load of glucose in a flavoured drink. Fasting values of >5.8 mmol/l or 2-hour values of >7.8 mmol/l require further testing.

INDICATIONS FOR GTT
Maternal weight >90th centile (>100 kg)
Previous big baby (>4.5 kg)
A first degree relative with diabetes
Glycosuria
Once at <20 weeks
Twice at >20 weeks
Previous unexplained stillbirth or neonatal death
Polyhydramnios
Fetal macrosomia on ultrasound

Table 4.1 High-risk features for abnormal glucose tolerance in pregnancy.

Treatment

There is no consensus view on treatment except that oral hypoglycaemics are contra-indicated. The following outline is suggested:

• Home monitoring by means of BM Stix or an electronic glucose monitor.

• Fasting and 1 hour blood sugar after each meal on at least 2 days a week.

• No treatment required if the fasting blood sugar level is <5.5 mmol/l and the postprandial figures are <9 mmol/l.

• If higher levels are involved, the woman should start a simple carbohydrate-restricted diet. In addition to checking her blood sugars twice a week, also test her urine for ketones.

• If the simple diet does not achieve the required blood sugar levels, a twice daily regimen of medium- and short-acting insulin.

• If ketosis occurs the diet should be relaxed and start insulin.

• Ultrasound scan for fetal growth and amniotic fluid volume at least monthly.

• If no evidence of excessive fetal growth, spontaneous labour can be awaited up to 42 weeks' gestation. Women with macrosomic fetuses shown on ultrasound should probably be induced at 38–39 weeks' gestation.

• Control of blood sugar in labour is important. Those on insulin antenatally should have the same i.v. glucose and insulin regimen as insulin-dependent diabetics.

• With the delivery of the placenta, the insulin requirements disappear.

• There is evidence that women who have gestational diabetes have about a 40% chance of becoming diabetic in the long term, the risk doubling if the woman is obese. In the latter case, once breast feeding is ceased, the woman is given strict dietary advice and advised to lose weight.

• Gestational diabetes usually recurs in future pregnancies but this is not inevitable.

Abdominal pain in pregnancy

Diagnosis depends mostly on history and examination with very few investigations helping.

EARLY PREGNANCY

Pelvic causes

I   Miscarriage:
   • Spontaneous: pain with contractions.

- Induced: pain with sepsis.
2 Retroversion and impaction of uterus.
- Pain from trapped bladder and retention of urine.
3 Fibroids.
- Pain from red degeneration — most common in mid-trimester.
4 Ovarian cysts.
- Pain from: rupture, twisting, or bleeding into cyst.
5 Ectopic pregnancy.
- Pain from: stretch, leak of blood from ostium of tube, or rupture.
6 Round ligament stretch.
- Pain from tension or haematoma.

Extrapelvic causes
1 Vomiting in pregnancy.
- Pain from abdominal wall muscle overstretch.
2 Urinary infection.
- Pain from bladder irritation and back pressure on kidney.
3 Appendicitis (Box 4.7).
- Pain from: peritoneal irritation, peritonitis, or rupture.

LATE PREGNANCY

Pelvic causes
1 Labour.
- Pain from myometrial contractions.
2 Hydramnios.
- Pain from stretch.
3 Abruptio placentae.
- Pain from myometrial damage and stretch.
4 Ruptured uterus.
- Pain from muscle damage or peritoneal involvement.

APPENDICITIS IN PREGNANCY

1 Underdiagnosed because it is not considered.
2 Undertreated due to fear of abdominal operations in pregnancy
3 Appendix pushed out of right iliac fossa and so general abdominal organ
4 Cortisol levels high, therefore poor inflammatory response
5 Omentum does not wall off inflamed organ.

Box 4.7 Reasons why appendicitis is a serious concern in pregnancy.

Extrapelvic causes

1 Rectus haematoma.
   - Pain from muscle stretch and irritation of tissues by blood.
2 Fulminating pre-eclampsia.
   - Pain from stretch of peritoneum over swollen liver.
3 Cholecystitis.
   - Pain from gall bladder stretch and inflammation.
4 Peptic ulcer.
   - Pain from associated gastritis and acid irritation of submucosal tissues.
5 Appendicitis — as before.
6 Pyelonephritis.
   - Pain from inflammation of pelvis or kidney.
7 Ureteric stone.
   - Pain from renal colic due to obstruction.

MANAGEMENT OF ABDOMINAL PAIN

- Make diagnosis accurately from history and examination and act soon to reduce morbidity.
- Use ultrasound with vaginal probe if considered helpful.
- Be prepared to use a laparoscope especially in early pregnancy.
- Do not consider laparotomy to be forbidden in pregnancy.
- A pregnancy in a woman with an intra-abdominal inflammatory disease will not be harmed by proper surgical treatment. The fetus is more likely to be damaged if the proper operation is delayed.

Infections in pregnancy

Any infection producing a pyrexia may cause miscarriage or preterm labour.

Two groups of infections are particularly important in pregnancy:

1 Genital tract infections.
2 Infections which cross the placenta.

GENITAL TRACT INFECTIONS

Syphilis

All pregnant women are still screened for syphilis because, while the disease is rare, appropriate treatment can prevent congenital syphilis. Treponemas readily cross the placenta from at least 10 weeks onwards.

Serological tests

These fall into two groups:

1 *Non-specific tests.*
   - The Wassermann reaction (WR).
   - The Venereal Disease Research Laboratory (VDRL) slide test.
   - The rapid plasma reagin (RPR) card test.

   False-positive tests may be seen with: chronic inflammatory diseases, yaws, narcotic abuse and pregnancy.

2 *Specific tests.*
   - The *Treponema pallidum* haemagglutination test (TPHA).
   - The fluorescent *Treponema* antibody test (FTA).

   These two tests are specific for *T. pallidum* and become positive some 2 weeks after the initial infection. They remain positive for ever once the patient has had the disease and do not produce biologically false-positive tests.

Effects on the fetus

1 Untreated early syphilis may result in neonatal death or stillbirth in 50%.

2 Congenital syphilis results in lasting neurological and skeletal damage.

Management

- *T. pallidum* is extremely sensitive to penicillin. Adequate treatment in early pregnancy protects the fetus. Even if the infection is only discovered in late pregnancy, treatment should still be given.
- Penicillin 1.2 mega-units i.m. for 10 days.
- Pregnant women who are sensitive to penicillin should be given erythromycin 500 mg orally every 6 hours for 15 days.
- The woman should be followed by the genitourinary physicians who should also contact her sexual partners.

Gonorrhoea

Neisseria gonorrhoeae is a Gram-negative, intracellular diplococcal organism.

Spread

- Gonorrhoea affects the endocervix, the urethra and possibly the rectum.
- Although gonorrhoea does not cross the placenta, it causes ophthalmia neonatorum if the baby is infected passing through the cervix at delivery.

Diagnosis
• Swabs should be taken from the endocervix and the urethra in suspected cases.
• Transport them to the laboratory in a suitable medium such as Stuart's medium.

Treatment
• Ampicillin 3 g plus probenecid 1 g in a single oral dose.
• In women who are penicillin-sensitive or if the *Gonococcus* species is resistant to penicillin, then ceftrioxone 250 mg i.m. should be used.

Trichomonas
A flagellate organism causing an intensely itchy, green-coloured, offensive, frothy discharge, occasionally bloodstained.

Diagnosis
• Microscopy with hanging drop of saline showing flagellated organisms moving rapidly.

Treatment
Oral metronidazole 200 mg 3 times/day for 7 days, for both the woman and her partner.
• Metronidazole may have an Antabuse-like effect so that patients should be advised not to drink alcohol.
• The fetus is very rarely affected by the presence of *Trichomonas*.

Candidiasis
Candida albicans is found in the mouth and gut of many. About 10% of non-pregnant and 40% of pregnant women have asymptomatic vaginal colonization.

Symptoms
• May cause intense vulval and vaginal pruritis, a discharge, or bleeding.

Diagnosis
• Causes thick white adherant plaques on the vaginal or cervical epithelium.
• Swabs should be taken for culture.

Treatment
• A single 500 mg Canesten pessary will cure most women.

- Resistant cases may need mechanical douching to remove organic material and then repeat the chemotherapy.

Herpes genitalis

Herpes simplex virus (HSV) is a large DNA virus. It enters a mucocutaneous surface, then migrates along nerves; it may undergo a latent phase in which it is resident in a ganglion.

Symptoms
- The first attack of herpes genitalis is usually acutely painful.
- Vesicles break down to form shallow ulcers on the cervix, labia, perineum or the perianal areas.
- There is inguinal lymphadenopathy.
- Recurrent attacks are less severe; many get warning symptoms of a tingling sensation in the affected area.

Diagnosis
- The lesions are usually clinically obvious.
- Ulcers should be scraped and sent for viral identification.

Effect on the newborn
- Herpes neonatorum may kill up to 50% of those with encephalitis but it is rare. A third of those remaining will have some residual neurological damage.
- The infection is acquired during the process of delivery or by ascending infection if the membranes have been ruptured for more than 4 hours.

Treatment
- Active infection in late pregnancy or early labour should lead to Caesarean section to avoid herpes neonatorum.
- Acyclovir is used with caution in pregnancy. Local attacks of herpes genitalis in the mother should be treated symptomatically.
- Acyclovir is used widely for the infant with herpes infection.

VAGINAL STREPTOCOCCAL INFECTIONS

β-haemolytic streptococcal infections may cause:

1 Preterm rupture of the membranes and preterm labour.
2 Severe postpartum sepsis, particularly following Caesarean section.
3 Overwhelming neonatal sepsis that may lead to death.
- About 1 : 5 women will carry group B streptococci in the vagina. About 1 : 50 women will give birth to an infected infant and about a third of these could die from overwhelming sepsis.

- Screening all pregnant women for the infection is not practical.
- All women presenting with preterm rupture of the membranes should have a sample of the amniotic fluid sent to identify the organism. If present, the baby should be delivered immediately.
- A woman who has lost a previous baby from overwhelming streptococcal infection should be given prophylactic i.v. ampicillin during labour.

LISTERIOSIS

Between 1% and 5% of pregnant women will carry *Listeria monocytogenes* in the rectum. The organism may in addition be acquired in pregnancy from eating unpasteurized cheese and from cooked meats. It may produce the following symptoms:

- Maternal diarrhoea accompanied by a pyrexia.
- Premature labour.

Listeriosis septicaemia of preterm infant acquired at birth may be rapidly fatal and may occur in the presence of few symptoms in the mother.

Treatment

Ampicillin i.v.

INFECTIONS THAT CROSS THE PLACENTA

The placenta acts as an efficient barrier against some infections in the mother. The following, however, are not uncommonly found in pregnant women and often cause serious consequences to the fetus:

- Syphilis (see p. 121).
- Rubella.
- Cytomegalovirus.
- Toxoplasmosis.
- Human immunodeficiency virus (HIV).
- Parvovirus.

Rubella

The widespread policy of vaccinating schoolgirls and more recently all children means that German measles (rubella) is becoming rarer. All pregnant women are tested for the levels of rubella antibodies at the antenatal clinic; if they are seronegative, they are vaccinated in the puerperium.

Rubella rapidly crosses the placenta and may cause:

- Mental retardation and microcephaly.
- Cataract.
- Congenital heart disease.
- Deafness.

- Hepatosplenomegaly with thrombocytopenia if the mother is infected in the last half of the pregnancy.

Women suspected of having acquired rubella in early pregnancy should have a rubella-specific IgM test. If positive, then the options available are:

1   Termination of pregnancy. This applies particularly if the primary infection was less than 10 weeks' gestation as more than half of the babies will be affected.

2   A chorionic villus sample. Electron microscopy and modern immune methods may be able to determine if the virus has crossed the placenta. This test can be performed from 8–11 weeks' gestation.

3   A fetal blood sample at 18–20 weeks' gestation (cordocentesis) to determine if the fetus is IgM-positive for rubella. If negative, the patient can be reassured. If positive, it confirms that the fetus has been infected but does not guarantee that it is affected. Most would ask for a termination of pregnancy on these grounds.

Cytomegalovirus (CMV)

CMV infection is now the most common perinatal infection in both the UK and USA. The most serious manifestations associated with primary maternal infection include:

- Stillbirth.
- Hepatosplenomegaly and jaundice.
- Thrombocytopenia.
- Microcephaly.
- Chorioretinitis.
  CMV may be acquired:
- In childhood from other children's saliva, tears, urine or stool.
- As an adult by sexual contact or blood transfusions.
- In the perinatal period by direct transmission across the placenta.

By the time pregnancy occurs, about 75% of women will be immune to CMV. Of women who acquire CMV in pregnancy, some 5% have a seriously damaged infant. Unlike rubella, there is no vaccination against the disease.

If the disease is suspected, it can be confirmed by looking for the IgM specific to CMV. Transplacental passage is not inevitable and the organism may be sought in the fetus by means of chorionic villus sample or fetal blood sample (see rubella).

Toxoplasmosis

Toxoplasma gondii comes from parasites in cats' intestines. Human infection occurs as a result of eating poorly cooked meats that contain tissue cysts or which have been exposed to infected cat faeces. Infection readily crosses the placenta. In the mother, it may be asymptomatic, or produce a glandular fever-like illness. Transplacental infection may cause:

- Microcephaly or hydrocephaly.
- Cerebral calcification leading to epilepsy and cerebral damage.
- Chorioretinitis.

The disease is diagnosed in the mother by finding an IgM specifically against toxoplasmosis. The mother can be treated by spiromycin to prevent further transplacental passage of the organism. Fetal infection may be diagnosed by means of fetal blood sampling and the search for specific IgM.

There is treatment available for the fetus but many women are offered a termination if their fetuses are infected.

Human immunodeficiency virus (HIV)

History

HIV is a retrovirus discovered in the 1980s. It affects the human, in some cases going on to the acquired immunodeficiency syndrome (AIDS). It attacks the helper subset of T lymphocytes and also other cells in the blood, alveoli and brain.

In Europe, anal intercourse is the commonest factor of spread.

The use of shared needles in i.v. drug abuse is another means of spreading the virus from an infected person. Blood transfusion may allow infection by the virus but in the UK all donor blood is screened for HIV. This is not so in all countries.

There is evidence in Britain that heterosexual transmission is increasing. Anonymous testing at antenatal clinics has shown HIV-positive women occur as commonly as 1 : 200 in the large towns, although this is much less frequent outside London and Edinburgh.

In pregnancy

Pregnancy may allow mild immunosuppression of the T cell type leading to a theoretical fear of exacerbation of HIV illness in pregnancy. This has not been borne out in clinical practice.

The fetus can be infected antenatally by the passage of HIV across the placenta. About 15% of babies born to mothers who are HIV-positive will remain HIV-positive at 6 months of age. It is estimated that 50% of these fetuses infected *in utero* will be dead from AIDS by 2 years.

- Women in high-risk groups (see p. 35) should be offered HIV testing after appropriate counselling.
- HIV can be isolated from cervical secretions and therefore the baby may be infected at birth. Antenatal infection is more likely so the method

of delivery does not influence infection. HIV may be passed in breast milk but this is doubtful.

• There is little evidence that asymptomatic HIV infection has any significant affect on pregnancy complications or the long-term outcome of women who are HIV-positive.

• Women who are HIV-positive need special care in the antenatal clinic, at delivery and in the puerperium, especially as they have major psychosocial problems.

• It is worth treating an HIV-positive woman in pregnancy with Zidovudine (Retrovir) because it passes to the fetus and greatly reduces the risks of HIV infection in the newborn.

• The risk of health workers acquiring infection is small if extra barrier precautions are adopted.

• Knowledge of the HIV status of newborn babies of high-risk women is essential in planning their vaccination policy against other infections. Vaccination with live attenuated vaccines should be avoided.

Hepatitis B

Hepatitis B virus is transmitted by contaminated blood products and occasionally by sexual intercourse. Transplacental rates of transmission are low amongst Europeans (<5%) but higher amongst Asians (40–90%).

The baby may be born apparently normal but develop hepatitis problems later. Rates may be reduced by both passive immunization with hepatitis B IgG and active immunization with hepatitis B vaccine.

The delivery presents problems to the staff because her blood and body products may contain live vaccine. In consequence, extra barrier precautions are taken.

Uterine conditions in pregnancy

RETROVERSION

Retroversion is the normal position of the uterus in 20% of women. If pregnancy occurs in a retroverted uterus:

• It usually comes upright as it enlarges.

• If tethered in the pouch of Douglas by old adhesions, it may enlarge by anterior sacculation.

• If the uterus is tethered it may grow and impact below the promontory of the sacrum. Growth can continue for a short time but soon there is:

  • Backache from pressure on the sacral peritoneum.

• Retention of urine from stretching of urethra by displacement of bladder into abdomen.

Unless this is relieved, the pregnancy will abort.

Management

1   Bed rest, with patient spending much time on her stomach.

2   Indwelling catheter and continuous bladder drainage.

3   Uterus often slides up into the abdomen. Once up, it will not go back so no pessary required.

CONGENITAL ABNORMALITIES OF UTERUS

Genital tract formed by fusion of two Mullerian ducts (Fig. 4.2a). Adjacent walls absorbed away at lower end (Fig. 4.2b) leaving a single lumen to the vagina, cervix and uterus but twin Fallopian tubes at upper end (Fig. 4.2c). Abnormal formation may be caused by:

• Only one Mullerian duct leading to uterus unicollis.

• Varying degrees of incomplete absorption of common walls (Fig. 4.3). Either can lead to:

1   Infertility.

2   Abortion.

3   Persistent malpresentations, especially transverse lie.

4   Dysfunction of myometrium, leading to incoordinate uterine action.

5   Obstructed labour (very rare).

6   PPH.

Management

1   Expect a normal delivery for often the non-pregnant half of the uterus rides up in late pregnancy and is no problem.

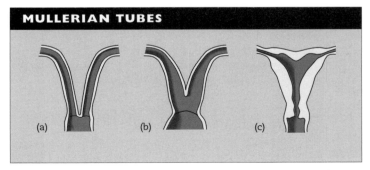

MULLERIAN TUBES

(a)   (b)   (c)

Fig. 4.2 Development of the female genital tract from two Mullerian tubes (see text).

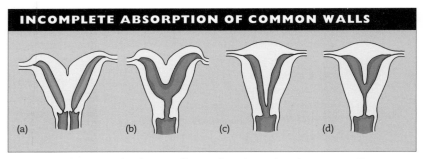

Fig. 4.3 Varying degrees of incomplete absorption of common walls.
(a) Double uterus, double cervix, vagina septum. (b) Double uterus, single
cervix. (c) Septate uterus. (d) Subseptate uterus.

2   If persistent transverse lie, Caesarean section. It is probably better to
do a classical approach and not a lower segment one for the latter could
give the operator no access to any part of the fetus which could be
delivered.

3   If vaginal septum ahead of presenting part, wait until second stage of
labour. When septum is maximally stretched by descending presenting
part, clamp and cut under local anaesthesia. This is always a much easier
and a less bloody operation than expected.

Pelvic tumours

FIBROIDS

Seen more commonly in the pregnancy age group among black women.

Diagnosis
Firm bosselated swellings detected usually in early pregnancy. Later they
soften and are difficult to locate. Ultrasound can usually detect fibroids.

Complications
I   Miscarriage.
2   Pressure:
   • On pelvic wall veins (oedema of legs).
   • On bladder (increased frequency).
3   Red degeneration:
   • Venous blood supply may be cut off and fibroid becomes stuffed with
   blood. Local pain and tenderness.
   • If diagnosed correctly, analgesia and bed rest allows resolution.

- If in doubt, perform laparotomy to check. If red degeneration seen, leave alone. Myomectomy during pregnancy is a very bloody operation.

4 Malpresentation:
- Oblique or transverse lie may persist because of position of fibroids.

5 Obstruction to labour:
- Very rarely happens, because lower uterine fibroids usually ride up into the abdomen when lower segment is formed and stretched.
- If cervical fibroids obstruct, Caesarean section must be performed but do not do myomectomy at the same time because of bleeding.

6 Dysfunction:
- Masses of fibrous tissue distort the smooth transmission of contractile impulses over uterus.

Re-examine woman 6 months after pregnancy. Most fibroids will have shrunk so much as not to require surgery.

OVARIAN CYSTS
In pregnancy:
- Corpus luteal cysts: 70%.
- Benign mucous or serous cystadenoma: 20%.
- Dermoid cyst: 5%.
- Malignant tumour: 1%.

Diagnosis
Mobile mass alongside or displacing uterus in early pregnancy. Ultrasound can usually help diagnosis.

Complications
1 Rupture of cyst.
2 Torsion of cyst.
3 Bleeding into cyst.
4 Obstruction in labour (rare).

Management
If any cyst over 10 cm diameter is detected, it should be removed. Try to do this in the middle trimester of pregnancy. Excise because:
- It may be malignant.
- It may undergo any of the above complications in labour or the puerperium.

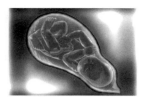

Physiology and Management of Normal Labour

The word labour is derived from the Latin word, *labor*, which means work. Labour is the act of expulsion of the fetus and placenta from the uterus and is traditionally divided into three successive stages. These stages are unequal in length (Fig. 5.1).

STAGES

The dilatation stage (first stage)

This is from the onset of labour until the cervix is fully dilated. More recently it has been divided into two phases:

1 The *latent phase*: the phase of effacement of the cervix.
2 The *active phase*: the phase of active cervical dilatation.

The expulsive stage (second stage)

This is from full cervical dilatation to complete expulsion of the baby.

The placental stage (third stage)

This is the time from expulsion of the baby until the expulsion of the placenta and membranes.

CHANGES IN PELVIC ORGANS DURING LABOUR

1 The cervix becomes effaced and dilates fully.
2 The uterus and vagina become one elongated tube.
3 The muscles of the pelvic floor and perineum are stretched backwards.
4 The bladder is pulled up becoming an abdominal organ and the urethra is lengthened.
5 The bowel is compressed.

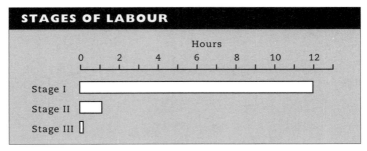

Fig. 5.1 Average length of stages of labour in a nullipara.

UTERINE ACTION

The fetus is propelled down the birth canal by the action of the uterine muscle (myometrium). Normal uterine activity is fundally dominant, so that waves of contraction pass down from the regions of the cornua to the lower uterine segment.

During labour, contractions increase in frequency and strength. Contractions are painful and this is unusual compared with other physiological muscle contractions. The cause of this may be due to:
• Hypoxia in the muscles because of the strength and duration of the contraction.
•   Compression of the nerve endings in the myometrium.
•   Cervical stretch and dilatation.

It is likely that there are pacemakers that initiate contractions and these are thought to be in each cornu. Unlike the sinu-atrial node of the heart, however, the uterine pacemakers cannot be distinguished histologically from the surrounding myometrium.

Figure 5.2 illustrates the patterns of propagation of the uterine activity. Labour starts with contractions about one in every 20 minutes and in normal labour, these increase as frequently as one in every 3 minutes. The upper uterine segment contracts and retracts so that the lower segment and later, the cervix, is pulled over the baby's head rather like pulling on a polo-neck sweater.

Figure 5.3 illustrates the intrauterine pressures that are achieved during normal labour.

MECHANISM OF LABOUR

In humans, the precise mechanism that causes labour is unknown. The following facts are accepted:

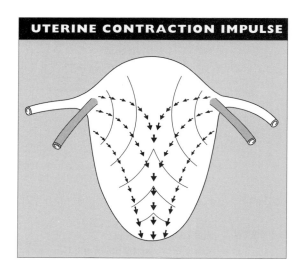

Fig. 5.2 Patterns of propagation of uterine contraction impulse.

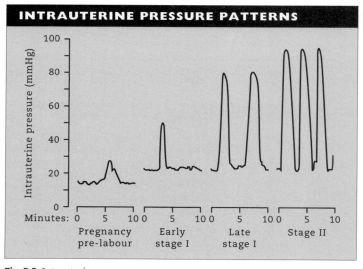

Fig. 5.3 Intrauterine pressure patterns.

- Oestrogens increase uterine muscle activity whilst progesterone suppresses it.
- In late pregnancy the fetal adrenal glands produce much more dehydro-epiandrosterone sulphate (DHEAS) which is converted by the placenta into oestrogen. This encourages uterine contractions.

• The decidua releases prostaglandins. Hypoxia of the decidua is thought to cause the start of labour. Released prostaglandins (PG) are mainly PGE_2 and $PGF_{2\alpha}$. Such PGs cause minor uterine contractions which result in further hypoxia of the decidua and a vicious circle is started.

• The final common pathway for a contraction is an increase in the cytosol-free calcium which causes a combination of actin and myosin. This is common to all involuntary muscle contractions.

• Oxytocin, released from the posterior pituitary, cannot be detected in the blood in early normal labour. The release of oxytocin is dependent upon a monosynaptic reflex, initiated when the presenting part presses on the pelvic floor.

The uterus in the first stage

1   Uterine muscle fibres contract and retract, so they do not return to their original length after contraction but remain shorter (Fig. 5.4).

2   There is a heaping up and thickening of the upper uterine segment while the lower uterine segment becomes thinner and stretched.

3   The cervix is pulled up and the canal is effaced; its length diminishes.

4   With further contractions, the cervix is pulled open and the os is dilated.

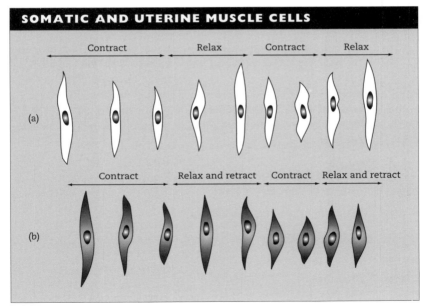

Fig. 5.4 (a) Somatic muscle cell contracting and relaxing. (b) Uterine muscle cell contracting and retracting.

These changes often start with the painless Braxton Hicks' contractions of late pregnancy so that by the beginning of labour the cervix is often already partially effaced and dilated. This is seen more frequently in multiparous women.

The uterus in the second stage

1   An increase in uterine length and a diminution in the anteroposterior and transverse diameters because of:
- Pulling up of the lower segment.
- Straightening out of the fetus.

2   The fetal head is forced into the upper vagina which now forms a continuous tube with the uterus and a fully effaced cervix.

3   As well as uterine contractions, expulsive efforts are made by the mother using:
- The abdominal wall muscles.
- The diaphragm, fixed by holding the breath, thus raising the intra-abdominal pressure.

4   Voluntary efforts are not essential for paraplegic women and those with epidural analgesia can have normal deliveries but they are instinctive, very satisfying to the woman and assist a delivery.

The uterus in the third stage

1   The uterine muscle contracts and constricts the blood vessels passing between the fibres, thus preventing excessive bleeding.

2   The placenta separates at the delivery of the fetus when the uterus sharply contracts in size. During pregnancy and most of the labour the placental bed and the placenta are roughly the same size. With the fetus removed, the area of the placental bed is reduced to about half that of the placental (Fig. 5.5). The placenta is therefore sheared off and is finally expelled from the uterus by contractions passing down into the lower segment.

The signs of descent of the placenta in the uterus are:
- The uterus becomes hard.
- The umbilical cord lengthens.
- There is a show of blood.

Management of normal labour

Diagnosis of labour

The onset of labour is defined as regular painful uterine contractions that

PLACENTAL SEPARATION

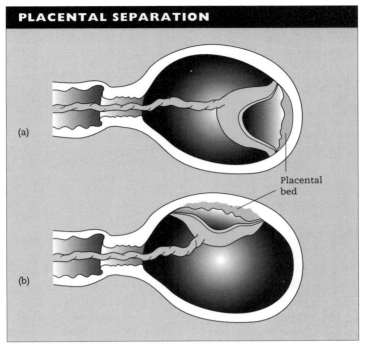

(a)

Placental bed

(b)

Fig. 5.5 (a) The commoner mechanism of placental separation in which the whole organ separates from its bed and balloons inside out into the uterine cavity. (b) Less common, the placenta separates at one side of the disc and is peeled off as the uterine muscle contracts and makes the placental bed much smaller in area.

cause cervical change. By its definition it often involves a retrospective diagnosis.

Admission

1 97% of women in the UK deliver in the hospital or general practice-run maternity unit.

2 Women should be advised to come into hospital when:
- Uterine contractions are occurring every 10 min.
- Their membranes rupture and amniotic fluid is released.

3 Assuming the woman had full antenatal care, on admission:
- A short history of labour is taken.
- A brief examination is performed including the following:
  (a) check the blood pressure;

(b) determine the lie and presentation of the fetus;

(c) determine the degree of engagement of the presenting part;

(d) perform a vaginal examination to assess the degree of efface-ment and dilatation of the cervix.

• The woman is offered a warm bath.

• The woman is offered a chance to open her bowels. If this is difficult, she may be offered some suppositories. Enemas are no longer given.

First stage of labour

Progress in labour is monitored by means of descent of the fetal head together with dilatation of the cervix. As little or nothing is known about the rate of cervical dilatation prior to admission to the labour ward, the partograph should be started on admission.

The partograph (Fig. 5.6), used by most maternity units, is an easy, graphical method of assessing the progress of labour and helps facilitate handover between midwives and doctors. It contains the following information:

1 A note of high-risk factors determined antenatally. These may be obstetric, paediatric or anaesthetic.

2 A record of the fetal heart rate. High-risk women will usually have continuous electronic fetal heart rate monitoring (EFM) by the car-diotocograph. Low-risk women usually have the fetal heart rate measured with a Pinard's stethoscope every 15 minutes, immediately following con-tractions. These records are plotted on the partograph.

3 The cervicogram: graphical record of the rate of fetal head descent during labour together with the rate of cervical dilatation.

4 Frequency, duration and strength of uterine contractions are recorded.

5 The state of the membranes and, if they are ruptured, the amniotic fluid colour.

6 The amount of maternal urine that is produced. Each specimen should be tested for ketones, protein and sugar.

7 A record of the drugs given, in particular analgesics.

8 Maternal blood pressure, pulse and temperature.

After the first examination the following should be plotted:

1 The amount of the fetal head that can be palpated per abdomen in terms of fifths of the head descent. Figure 5.7 illustrates the system of fifths.

2 The cervical dilatation (Fig. 5.8).

3 A partogram should then also be plotted. This may be one of a series of curves cut in a plastic overlay or it may be a straight line plotted at 1 cm/hour.

The level of descent of the presenting part should be checked and

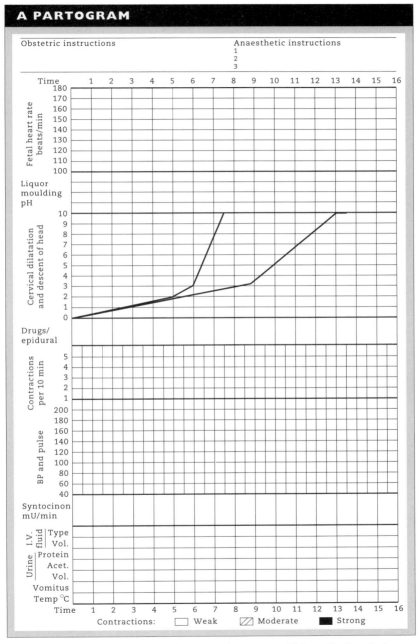

Fig. 5.6 A partogram used to assess the progress of labour. The lines in the cervical dilated section are the expected patterns of cervical dilatation in nulliparous and primiparous labour.

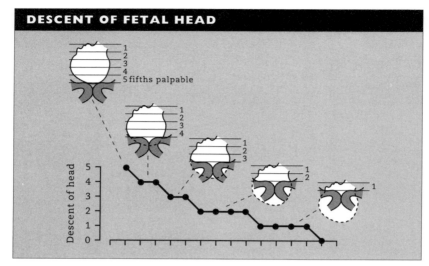

Fig. 5.7 Expected normal progress and descent of fetal head through pelvis.

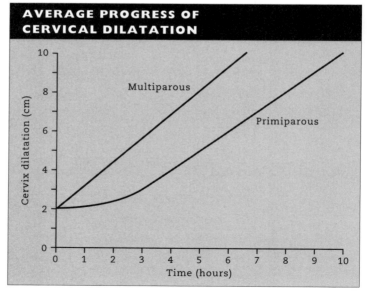

Fig. 5.8 The progress of cervical dilatation for multiparous and primiparous women.

plotted every hour, whilst vaginal examinations are performed every 3–4 hours. As long as the rate of cervical dilatation stays on or to the left of the nomogram, labour progress is considered to be normal.

Care of the patient
• The woman should not be left alone during labour. Ideally there should be a midwife present with her throughout the labour. In addition, many women choose to have their partner, companion or relative present.
• Analgesia should be given which is sufficient for the woman's need.
• She should be encouraged to pass urine frequently. If the bladder becomes palpable and the woman cannot void, she should be catheterized.
• As the stomach emptying time slows during labour, no heavy food should be given once contractions start but light snacks, soup or cool fluids are offered.

Second stage of labour
1 During the expulsive stage, the woman is encouraged to push with uterine contractions by taking a deep breath and holding it, putting her chin on her chest, and pulling on the backs of her knees. Effective pushing is hard to learn before the second stage of labour. Women usually manage to get two or three expulsive pushes during each uterine contraction.

2 Monitoring progress in the second stage of labour is difficult until the presenting part becomes visible.

3 Inhalation analgesia should be offered in the second stage of labour if the woman requires it. However, with organized pushing, many women do not require pain relief.

4 Episiotomies are no longer performed routinely but are indicated for the following reasons:
  • Fetal distress.
  • Most operative vaginal deliveries.
  • The presence of a rigid perineum which, in the opinion of the midwife, is delaying delivery.
  • If an experienced midwife believes that there is going to be a major perineal tear.
  Minor tears often do not need suturing and heal well.

5 If an episiotomy is to be performed, local anaesthetic (lignocaine 1% plain) is injected into the subcutaneous tissues of the vagina and perineum as the head distends the perineum. Just prior to crowning, a right mediolateral episiotomy is usually performed with slow extension of the head the episiotomy does not extend.

6 When the head is delivered, it is allowed to rotate (restitute) and then lateral traction is applied in the direction of the mother's anus which allows the birth of the fetal anterior shoulder.

7   At this stage, 0.5 mg of Syntometrine is injected i.m. into the mother's thigh to aid with delivery of the placenta.

8   The baby's head is then raised towards the mother's abdomen so the posterior shoulder passes over the perineum and the rest of the baby usually then slips out.

9   The baby's mouth and then the nasal passages are usually sucked free of mucus with a mechanical mucus extractor. The mouth should be cleared before the nose as aspirating the nose often causes the baby to inhale.

10   The umbilical cord is then clamped twice, and divided between the clamps. In developed countries, hospital units now use disposable plastic umbilical clamps.

11   The baby usually starts breathing within 1 minute of delivery. The baby may be given to the mother immediately if she so wishes but should be wrapped in a prewarmed blanket first.

Third stage of labour

1   Active management of the third stage of labour starts with the injection of Syntometrine (a mixture of ergometrine 0.5 mg and Syntocinon 5 i.u.) with the delivery of the anterior shoulder of the infant. Signs of placental separation are no longer awaited before applying controlled cord traction.

2   The operator's left hand is placed above the symphysis pubis and guards the front wall of the fundus of the uterus to prevent uterine inversion.

3   The umbilical cord is grasped in the operator's right hand and steady traction is applied until the placenta is delivered down into the vagina. A kidney dish is then placed under the patient's perineum, held in the operator's left hand and the placenta is fully delivered into the dish.

4   The membranes usually follow the placenta and can be removed by gentle rotation of the placenta. It allows them to peel off the uterus.

5   The placenta and membranes should then be checked for completeness.

6   Blood loss should be estimated and is usually between 100 and 300 ml.

7   Any tear or episiotomy should be carefully repaired with absorbable sutures such as Vicryl under local anaesthetic (Fig. 5.9).

Pain relief in labour

- Labour is usually painful. Relief of pain is better given before the woman feels the pain of the contractions.
- Careful timing of analgesia is as important as correct dosage.

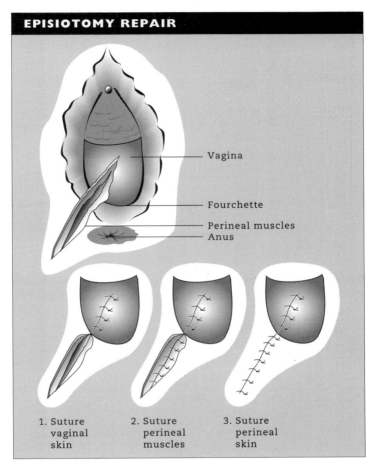

Fig. 5.9 Repair of an episiotomy.

ANALGESIA

The reduction of pain by reducing cortical sensitivity.

Drugs by inhalation

Nitrous oxide

This can be self-administered, pre-mixed with O_2 (50% of each); it comes in blue and white quartered cylinders for use with Entonox machines. Nitrous oxide and air mixtures used to be given with light portable equipment but this is not advised for it reduces the O_2 available. Inhalation should start as the contraction is felt and before the woman feels pain (Fig. 5.10) for it takes some seconds to work.

Drugs by other routes

Pethidine

- Synthetic analgesic with antispasmodic action on smooth muscle. Very useful for labour.
- Dose: 50–150 mg i.m.;
    50–100 mg i.v. (slowly, for it can cause nausea).

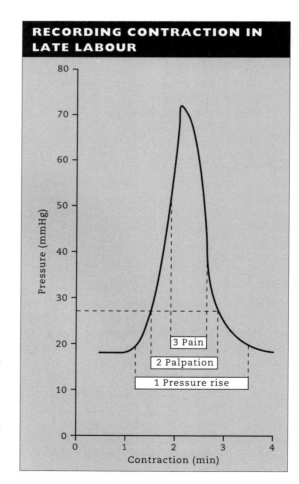

Fig. 5.10 Pressure recording of contraction in late labour: (1) tocograph pressure readings show activity for 2 minutes; (2) clinical abdominal palpation diagnosis shows contraction for 1 minute; (3) pain is felt by the woman for 45 seconds.

• Use in first stage. Try to avoid giving within 2 hours of expected delivery if possible because of depression of neonatal respiration.
• Can cause drop of maternal blood pressure especially when combined with antiemetic.

Morphine

• An alkaloid of opium. Stronger analgesic but no antispasmodic action. Well used for the dull pains of occipitoposterior positions and long labours.
• Dose: 10 mg i.m.
• Morphine depresses the neonatal respiratory centre, and should be avoided for 2 hours before delivery if possible.
• May cause maternal vomiting (about 15%) so give with an anti-emetic (e.g. Phenergan 25 mg or Fentazin 5 mg).

Diamorphine (heroin)

• Very powerful opiate. Good for anxious mother or long labour.
• Dose: 5–10 mg i.m.
• Depresses neonatal respiratory centre if given within 3–4 hours.
• Still used a lot in Scotland and north of England.

Meptazinol (Meptid)

• Strong analgesic with less depressive action on respiration.
• Dose: 100–150 mg up to 2 hours.

Aspirin

• Salicylate: a mild analgesic. Occasionally used in very early labour.
• Dose: 300–600 mg orally.
• Can cause haematemesis and not very powerful.

Note
Barbiturates, tranquillizers and sedatives given in labour are *not* analgesics. They often potentiate analgesics and help progress by their own properties.

NON-DRUG ANALGESIA

Increasing numbers of women are turning to non-pharmacological methods of pain relief. Pain is such a subjective symptom that anything that helps a woman and does not put her or her fetus at increased risk should be explored. Maybe these methods cause the release of endorphins and so postpone the need for more formal analgesia; this reduces the total dose, giving the woman a greater sense of self-participation.

Hypnosis

If both woman and attendant are properly trained, this can give good pain relief. It is expensive on attendant's time and only works for susceptible women. If it works, it is very safe for the fetus.

Transcutaneous nerve stimulation

Transcutaneous nerve stimulation provides small pulses of electrical vibration to the muscles of the lower back, from a portable battery-driven pack. It provides distraction therapy and some women find it helpful in the early stages of labour. Even though it might not work for full labour, it could postpone the need for a stronger more depressing analgesia and so its use should be encouraged if women want to try it. However, labour ward staff must know how to work the machines and be sympathetic to their use.

ANAESTHESIA

Depression of the central or peripheral nervous system to prevent transmission and reception of painful impulses.

General

Total anaesthesia induced by injection (e.g. pentothal) and followed by inhalation (e.g. nitrous oxide or cyclopropane) results in an unconscious patient completely under the anaesthetist's control.

In labour one of the risks is regurgitation of acid stomach contents and their inhalation into the lungs producing aspiration pneumonia (Mendelson's syndrome). To avoid this:
- Have empty stomach—in labour do not have indigestable meals.
- If really necessary, ensure stomach empty—pass a tube.
- Reduce acidity of stomach contents—give sodium citrate (30 ml) or H_2 blocker, e.g. ranitidine.
- Pass cuffed endotracheal tube.
- Tilt head up for intubation and use cricoid pressure.
- Only skilled senior anaesthetists deal with women in labour.

General anaesthesia is useful for operations such as an emergency Caesarean section when speed is essential.

Regional

Nerve roots are blocked at their outflow.

Spinal

- Heavy nupercaine into subarachnoid space.
- Give at L3–4, put woman in head-up position.

- Blocks $T_{11}-S_1$.
- Used once only usually for operative procedures.
- Good anaesthetic used increasingly in UK for one off procedures, e.g. forceps.

Epidural block

- Xylocaine 1% or Marcain 0.25–0.5% through a cannula inserted into peridural fat. Affects nerve roots $T_{11}-S_4$.
- Pain relief rapid, lasting 2–3 hours.
- Repeated doses can be given; therefore used for pain relief in labour.
- Requires expertise of an anaesthetist to put it in the right place (Fig. 5.11).
- Loss of all sensation from the uterus means the woman needs help in the second stage to recognize uterine contractions.

Complications

- A serious complication of the epidural block is to puncture the dura and so unwittingly perform a spinal anaesthetic. This could lead to nerve blockage and stopping respiration if the anaesthetic agent flows up into

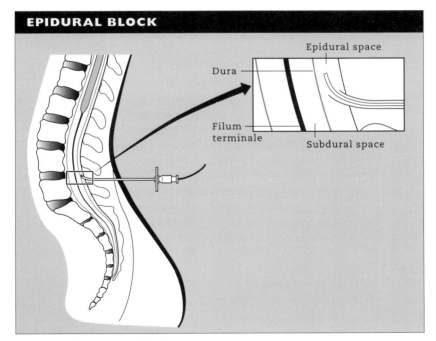

Fig. 5.11 An epidural block.

the thoracic region. Such a complication is watched for carefully by an experienced anaesthetist and can be dealt with.
• Dural tap in 1:500 cases with subsequent CSF leak.
• A rarer complication is infection which might enter through the skin to the peridural area.

Caudal block
• Localized epidural through sacral hiatus.
• Gives good anaesthesia for operative deliveries but only 80% effective.

Paracervical block
• Injection, into the base of the cardinal ligaments from lateral fornices of vagina of Xylocaine or Marcain affects most nerves leaving uterus. Can be repeated when relief wears off (2–4 hours).
• Good anaesthetic for later part of first stage of labour.

Local

Pudendal
• Block pudendal nerve with Xylocaine 0.5 or 1% in its two or three branches as it circumnavigates the ischial spine; given either through vagina or through perineal skin. Numbs the area on the left as shown in Fig. 5.12, but therefore needs a field block as well.

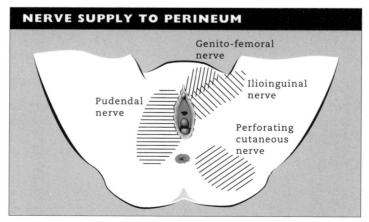

NERVE SUPPLY TO PERINEUM

Genito-femoral nerve

Ilioinguinal nerve

Pudendal nerve

Perforating cutaneous nerve

Fig. 5.12 The sensory nerve supply of the skin of the perineum. While the pudendal nerve principally supplies this area, other nerves are involved and need consideration in anaesthetizing the perineum locally.

- Used for outlet manipulations in the second stage of labour, e.g. easy forceps delivery.

Field block

A local infiltration of the nerve endings in the vulva and labia:
- Prior to episiotomy or its repair.
- As an adjunct to pudendal block to anaesthetize those areas not covered by the block.

Proper analgesia and anaesthesia in labour work best when the woman and her partner have been instructed antenatally and have had a chance to learn about the methods available. She should talk to other women who have benefited by analgesia. All this is then applied by sympathetic attendants who look to the needs of individual women and tailor the therapy to their needs, preferably preventing pain being felt rather than trying to remove it after it has arrived.

The fetus during labour

During labour the fetus descends and is delivered from the birth canal. The process is conventionally broken down into the series of mechanisms detailed below, which merge with each other and are inseparable.

Flexion

Uterine activity is fundally dominant; the line of force is down the fetal spine and at first this causes flexion of the fetal head. In many cases flexion occurs before labour starts as a result of Braxton Hicks' contractions. Following flexion the head engages when the presenting diameter passes through the pelvic brim. In most cases the head engages in the occipito-transverse position and in the majority of cases this is the right occipito-transverse position.

Descent

Further uterine activity causes the fetal head to descend through the pelvic brim to the mid-cavity.

Internal rotation

Due to the angle of inclination between the lumbar spine and the pelvis (about 135°), the fetal head engages in the pelvis with one parietal eminence lower than the other (asynclitism). The leading parietal eminence is then pushed into the pelvic floor with uterine contractions. When the uterus relaxes, the reaction from the pelvic floor muscles causes the fetal head to rotate until the head is no longer asynclitic. The head rotates from the right occipitotransverse position at engagement to become direct occipitoanterior (Fig. 5.13).

Further flexion

Further descent through the pelvis together with uterine contractions causes the fetal chin to be forced tightly up against the fetal chest. The fetal occiput comes to lie on the maternal symphysis pubis and the chin comes down to the lower part of the birth canal.

Extension

Further descent pushes the fetal head forward and gradual extension of the fetal head occurs distending the perineum. With further extension the widest diameter passes through the vulval introitus (crowning) and the head is born by extension at the fetal neck.

Restitution and internal rotation

As the head is born, the shoulders enter the maximum diameter (the transverse diameter) of the maternal pelvic inlet. As they descend through the canal, one shoulder leads because of the angle of inclination. This causes the shoulders to rotate (just as the head did in internal rotation) and, as they do so, the head rotates 90°. As the shoulders come to lie in the anteroposterior diameter behind the maternal symphysis pubis, the head rotates to lie in its usual alignment with the shoulders. Since the head is now outside the vulva, this is external rotation.

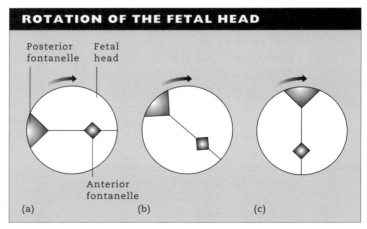

Fig. 5.13 Internal rotation of the fetus. (a) Inlet: right occipitotransverse position. (b) Mid-cavity: right occipitoanterior position. (c) Outlet: direct occipitoanterior position.

Delivery of the body

By lateral flexion of the fetal head, the anterior shoulder is made to slip under the pubis and is born. The posterior shoulder and the rest of the body follows usually very easily.

During each uterine contraction the maternal blood supply to the intervillous space is severely reduced and is often cut off. This reduces the fetal O_2 supply and allows less time for exchange of waste products from the fetus to the mother. Most normal fetuses can stand intermittent hypoxic ischaemia but preterm babies and those who are SGA may run into danger at this time. In consequence, the fetus often needs to be carefully monitored during labour.

MONITORING THE FETUS DURING LABOUR

There has been much recent controversy about the value of electronic fetal monitoring (EFM) in labour. There is probably no proven value for continuous EFM in low-risk pregnancies. Such women may have a short (20 minutes) cardiotocograph recording on admission to the labour ward and thereafter the fetal heart is listened to every 15 minutes with a Pinard stethoscope.

The following factors should be considered at high risk of hypoxia in labour and therefore should have continuous EFM:

- Preterm infants (less than 37 weeks' completed gestation).
- Fetuses that are or are suspected to be SGA.
- Multiple pregnancies.
- Breech presentations.
- Women with epidural analgesia.
- Women with Syntocinon augmentation of labour.
- Women who have been induced.
- Women who are hypertensive.
- Women with major medical disoders, including diabetes.
- Women who develop meconium staining of the amniotic fluid during the labour.
- Women who undergo a trial of uterine scar.
- If a fetal heart abnormality is recorded with the Pinard stethoscope.

Continuous electronic fetal heart rate monitoring

In all modern labour wards, this is performed with either:

1   An external fetal heart rate monitor with Doppler ultrasound echoing off movements of the fetal cardiac walls or the cardiac valves.

2   An electrode attached to the fetal scalp (Fig. 5.14) showing the fetal heart rate derived from the fetal ECG.

Either of these provides the fetal heart rate and this is recorded on a

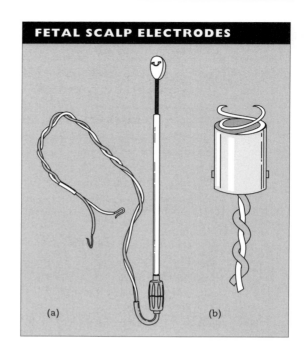

FETAL SCALP ELECTRODES

(a)   (b)

Fig. 5.14 Fetal scalp electrodes for (a) clipping onto or (b) screwing into the skin of the fetal presenting part thus providing electrical continuity.

continuous trace. In normal labour, this should be between 110 and 160 beats/minute. EFM is used as a screening test to detect those babies who are developing metabolic acidosis. The diagnostic test is to perform a fetal scalp sample and measure the scalp pH.

Changes in the fetal heart rate may be classified into two groups.

Alterations in baseline heart rate

1 A *fetal tachycardia*. Figure 5.15 demonstrates a fetal tachycardia of about 170 beats per min. The causes of this might be:

- A maternal tachycardia due to pyrexia, pain, fear or dehydration.
- Fetal hypoxia.

Management is to exclude or correct a maternal cause and, if the tachycardia persists, then a fetal blood sample should be performed.

2 A *baseline bradycardia*. Baseline bradycardias are uncommon and provided they are in the 110–120 beats/minute range and there is baseline variability they are not of serious significance (Fig. 5.16). Bradycardias of <110 beats/minute in labour are most commonly due to congenital heart block.

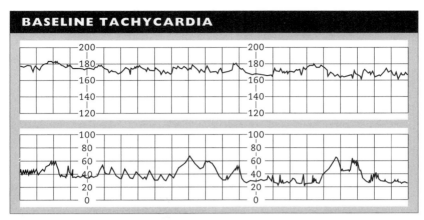

Fig. 5.15 A CTG demonstrating an uncomplicated, moderate, baseline tachycardia. The baseline is 170 beats/minute. The reduced variability is a feature of the tachycardia. This trace was due to a maternal pyrexia in labour consequent upon a urinary tract infection.

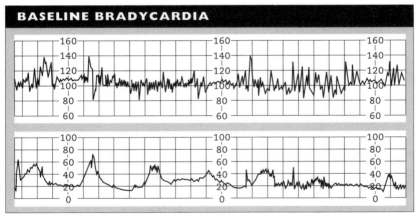

Fig. 5.16 A CTG demonstrating a moderate baseline bradycardia. The baseline is 100 beats/minute. No cause for this was found.

Baseline variability

Terminology in this area is difficult because of the way in which the machinery records the heart rate. Most external Doppler machines average every third beat and so the term beat-to-beat variation should be reserved for fetal heart rate traces that are obtained by fetal scalp electrodes.

The variation in fetal heart rate from one beat to the next (baseline variability) is due to the balance between the parasympathetic and the sympathetic nervous system. In normal labour this varies by 5–10 beats either side of the baseline. Accelerations (see Fig. 2.6) are intermittent periods in which the fetal heart rate is raised quite markedly above the baseline. They are a sign of fetal health.

The major variations of baseline variability are:

1 *Loss of baseline variability.* This is illustrated in Fig. 5.17 and may be caused by:

• Administration of drugs to the mother including pethidine, diazepam and many antihypertensive agents, especially β-blockers.

• Fetal hypoxia. In the absence of maternal drugs, loss of baseline variability should lead to a fetal blood sample.

2 *Increased baseline variability* (sinusoidal rhythm). This is illustrated in Fig. 5.18 and usually is of serious significance. The causes of it are as follows:

• Fetal asphyxia.

• Fetal anaemia, e.g. due to Rh incompatibility.

3 *Deceleration.* Decelerations are intermittent changes in the baseline and fall into four categories:

• Type I or early deceleration.

These are illustrated in Fig. 5.19 and are due to vagal stimulation following head compression as the fetus descends the birth canal. They usually have no significance and do not require a fetal blood sample unless the fetus is preterm.

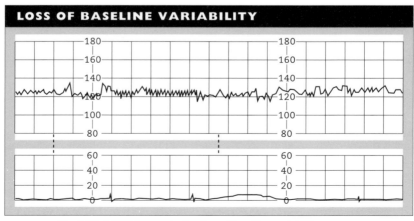

Fig. 5.17 A CTG demonstrating loss of baseline variability.

SINUSOIDAL RHYTHM

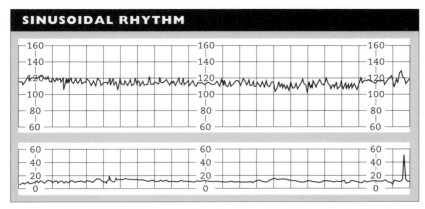

Fig. 5.18 A CTG demonstrating minor sinusoidal rhythm. The baseline is 110 beats/minute.

EARLY DECELERATION (TYPE I)

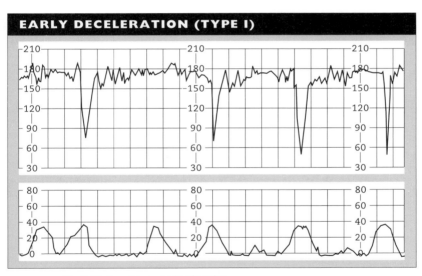

Fig. 5.19 Type I or early deceleration.

- Type II or late decelerations.

    These are illustrated in Fig. 5.20. They differ from type I decelerations in that they are U-shaped, start more than 30 seconds after the contraction has started and continue after the contraction has finished. They are thought to be metabolic in nature and always warrant a fetal blood sample.

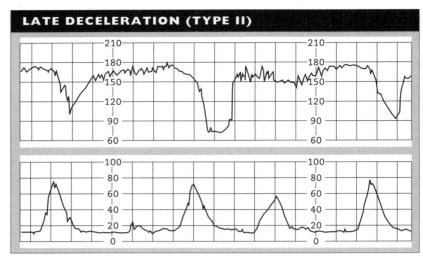

Fig. 5.20 Type II or late deceleration.

- Variable decelerations.

  These are also of two types:

  (a) *Isolated variable decelerations* (Fig. 5.21). These are commonly seen in labour following the use of a bed pan or after an epidural top-up. They may also result from umbilical cord compression and will usually disappear if the woman is turned on the other side. As long as the fetal heart rate trace returns to normal following the deceleration, the baby will not be asphyxiated and fetal blood sampling is not required.

  (b) *Recurrent variable decelerations* (Fig. 5.22). The important features to note are that the decelerations vary both within shape and in their relationship to the uterine contraction. The most common cause of these is cord compression. Either the cord is compressed between the presenting part and the pelvic side walls or the cord is around the fetal neck or a limb. They do not normally require a fetal blood sample but, if associated with meconium or a change in the baseline heart rate, one should be performed.

PASSAGE OF MECONIUM

Stimulation of the vagus *in utero* may cause the fetal gut to contract and the anal sphincter to relax such that meconium (fetal stool) is passed into the amniotic fluid. Meconium is the accumulation of swallowed cells in late

OXYTOCIN-INDUCED PROFOUND DECELERATION

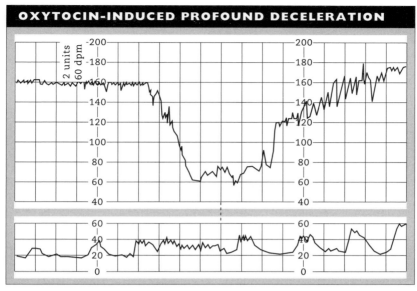

Fig. 5.21 Oxytocin-induced profound deceleration.

VARIABLE DECELERATIONS

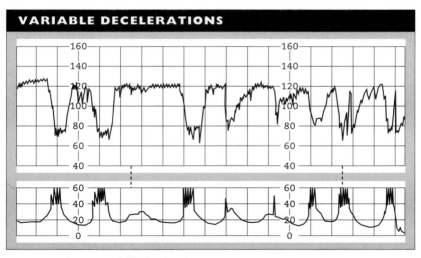

Fig. 5.22 Variable decelerations.

pregnancy with cells shed from the alimentary tract, all of which are stained with bile.

With a normal fetal heart rate trace, it is unlikely that the fetus is hypoxic and fetal blood sampling is not necessary. If the fetal heart rate trace is at all abnormal and meconium is passed, then it should be performed.

FETAL BLOOD SAMPLE

Fetal blood sampling is a diagnostic test for fetal acidosis. A bead of blood is taken from the fetal scalp and the pH and base deficit is measured.

During a uterine contraction:
- Maternal blood flow to the intervillous space is vastly reduced or may cease.
- Passage of O_2 from the mother to the fetus is reduced and thus the fetus may become hypoxic.
- The fetus withstands these periods of hypoxia by employing anaerobic metabolism. To do this, the fetus must mobilize glycogen from liver and muscle stores to produce glucose as an energy source.
- Anaerobic metabolism results in the production of large amounts of lactic acid and an increase in the arterial CO_2. In normal circumstances, the rise in arterial CO_2 is buffered, mostly by fetal Hb.
- Between contractions the lactic acid and the buffered CO_2 are passed back to the mother who excretes the latter by increasing her respiratory rate leading to a respiratory alkalosis.
- If glycogen stores are poor as in those who are preterm or those who are SGA, other sources of energy are required for anaerobic metabolism.

These produce more CO_2 and more lactic acid and thus fetal buffering systems become impaired. This results in a gradual fall of pH; the fetus demonstrates a metabolic acidosis.

If uterine activity is too frequent or sustained, then blood flow to the fetus may be impaired for a long space of time and this, again, will result in a metabolic acidosis with an increasing base deficit.

Figure 5.23 illustrates the mechanism by which the fetal scalp sample is acquired. The fetal scalp is punctured with a guarded blade and the blood is aspirated into a capillary tube.

The pH results are interpreted as follows:
- pH $>$ 7.25: normal.
- pH 7.20–7.25: pre-asphyxia.
- pH $<$ 7.20: asphyxia.
- Base deficit $<$ 6.0 mEq/l: normal.
- Base deficit 6.1–7.9 mEq/l: pre-asphyxia.
- Base deficit $>$ 8.0 mEq/l: asphyxia.

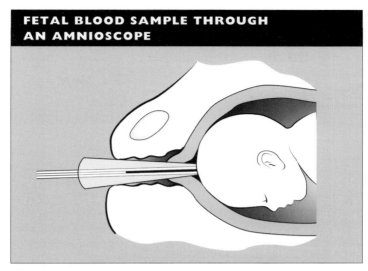

FETAL BLOOD SAMPLE THROUGH AN AMNIOSCOPE

Fig. 5.23 Fetal blood samples can be taken from the scalp through an amnioscope.

In obstetric practice it is common to use the term asphyxia but what is truly meant is a metabolic acidosis.

Any fetus who has a pH of <7.20 and a base deficit >8.0 mEq/l should be delivered immediately by the most appropriate route. Fetuses that demonstrate pre-asphyxia and are in the second stage may be allowed normal delivery only if this is imminent.

The scalp pH only reflects the state of the fetus at the time of the sample; the base deficit reflects a slower change, therefore is a longer predictor. If the fetal heart rate trace continues to be abnormal, then the fetal blood sample should be repeated hourly or the baby delivered.

The newborn after delivery

If a preterm or at-risk infant is about to be delivered, an experienced paediatrician should be on hand to provide appropriate resuscitation. As soon as the infant is born, assess its condition. A fuller analysis is in the Apgar score.

The three essential states may be:
- *Healthy*: pink; effective regular respiration.
- *Inadequate breathing*: irregular shallow or gasping respiration.
- *Terminal apnoea*: white; floppy; no attempt to breathe.

Healthy

    1   Do not suck out unless necessary.

    2   If upper airway contains meconium, blood or mucus, then laryngoscope infant and aspirate trachea and larynx under direct vision.

    3   Wrap in a blanket and hand to mother.

Inadequate breathing

    1   If not present, call paediatrician urgently. Carry out the following:

      • Give face mask O_2.

      • Gentle peripheral stimulation.

      • Oropharyngeal suction.

      • Dry and cover lower body with warm towels.

    2   If the infant does not respond to this by 1–1.5 minute (i.e. respiration not established and heart rate falling below 80 beats/minute) extend neck, hold jaw forward and apply face mask closely to face to obtain a tight seal and give intermittent positive-pressure ventilation (IPPV) through the mask, at about 30 breaths/minute, 100% O_2.

    3   If the infant still remains blue with inadequate respiration and a falling heart rate at 2.5–2 minute; laryngoscope, aspirate any mucus or meconium under direct vision and intubate. Give IPPV at pressures of 20 cmH$_2$O (maximum 30 cmH$_2$O) and a rate of 30/minute. Most infants will respond to this. Ensure meconium completely sucked out before IPPV.

    4   As soon as the infant improves with any of the above (i.e. heart rate 140 beats/minute, spontaneous respiration and pink in colour) remove endotracheal tube, watch for respiration to be established.

    5   Analgesics such as pethidine or morphine given to the mother late in labour can depress respiration in the infant. Once respiration has started but is not fully established Naloxone can be given at a dose of 10 µg/kg estimated weight i.v. or i.m. Do not give naloxone to baby of a drug-dependent mother as this may cause withdrawal, fits or death.

    6   There is no indication for analeptic drugs in the management of birth asphyxia.

    7   Preterm babies need intubation earlier than term babies.

    8   Do not perform IPPV with a mask on very small babies.

Terminal apnoea

    1   Do not delay resuscitation if, at this stage, the infant is pale, limp and apnoeic with a heart rate of less than 100.

    2   If not present, call paediatrician urgently.

    3   Laryngoscopy, aspirate under direct vision and intubate. Give IPPV rate 30/minute, 20–30 cmH$_2$O with 100% O_2.

    4   These infants may:

- Respond over 2–3 minutes.
- Require naloxone (if appropriate) to get spontaneous respiration established.
- Remain apnoeic — assume birth asphyxia likely and give sodium bicarbonate i.v. and adrenaline via endotracheal tube under supervision of paediatrician.

5 Get a cord blood estimate of pH and base deficit.

6 Admit to neonatal unit if:
- Poor response to resuscitation.
- Base deficit > 15 mEq/l

7 Let mother hold baby before transfer to neonatal unit.

Home deliveries

Until this century, the place of birth was most usually the home. Hospital deliveries started in the mid-eighteenth century for charitable reasons to help poor women with unsuitable conditions at home and the unmarried. It has grown gradually this century from 2% in 1900 to 98% in 1990.

Home deliveries had atrophied to about 1% by 1986, but are slightly increasing in this last decade to a provisional figure of almost 2% in 1994 (see Fig. 5.24).

The drift to hospitalization has occurred:

- As part of the fashion of using a hospital for medical affairs.

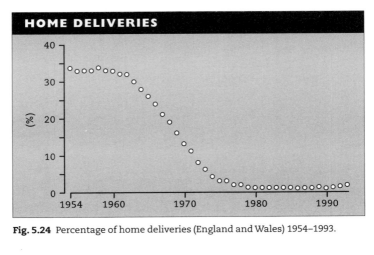

Fig. 5.24 Percentage of home deliveries (England and Wales) 1954–1993.

- For safety. In the isolation of the home, it would be difficult to care for an emergency:

    (a) PPH.

    (b) Delayed onset of baby breathing.

    Against this, the advantages of home delivery are:
- Familiar surroundings for the woman.
- More relaxation because of confidence at home.
- Probably would know the midwife who was delivering her.
- More family members could attend the birth and the immediate time afterwards.

The slight increase in home deliveries means that a community service must be kept going. Two midwives must attend each home delivery and these are usually of higher skills than those working in the hospitals. A general practitioner can be called in an emergency. If the woman has to be transferred to hospital, the use of an ambulance with paramedics, skilled in resuscitation, must be obtained.

The future of the hospital/domiciliary debate could be eased by:

- The use of a birthroom in the hospital, but away from the main Labour Ward. To here the community midwife can bring the woman in labour with her partner. If delivery is normal and all goes well, they can return home a few hours later and so have never really entered the hospital.
- Reduce the regimentation of hosptial.
- Reduce the noise of the wards.
- Provide clean wards, linen and lavatories.
- Get the woman back home early on day 1 or 2.
- Use of formal DOMINO services.
- Use of birth rooms.

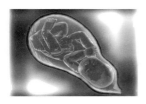

Pathology and Management of Abnormal Labour

Dysfunctional uterine action

Prolonged labour is rarely a primary uterine fault but is a result of relative or absolute cephalopelvic disproportion (CPD). The progress of labour should be monitored on a partogram. Figure 6.1 illustrates the normal rate of cervical dilatation from the start of labour. During the first 8 hours in primiparous women there is minimal change in the cervical dilatation but effacement occurs — the latent phase. Effacement is the taking up of the cervix, merging with the lower segment; eventually there is no length to the cervical canal.

Three abnormalities of labour may be recognized.

Prolonged latent phase

This is a rare abnormality and occurring almost exclusively in primigravidae. Figure 6.2 illustrates this together with the possible outcome. Aetiological factors are:

- The wrong diagnosis of labour.
- An abnormal or high presenting part.
- Premature rupture of the membranes.
- Idiopathic: cervical dystocia.
  (a) Primary. Failure of a ground substance of the cervix to soften in late pregnancy.
  (b) Secondary. Operations on the cervix causing fibrosis.

Management

1 Women who present with regular uterine activity should be assessed by bimanual vaginal examination; if the cervix is long and closed, they may

163

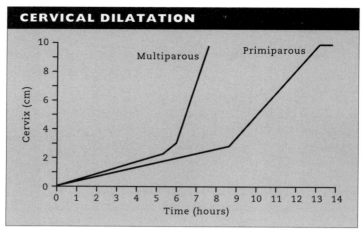

Fig. 6.1 Average rate of cervical dilatation in labour for multiparous and primiparous women.

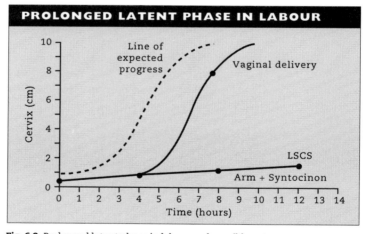

Fig. 6.2 Prolonged latent phase in labour and possible outcomes.

be in early or in false labour. A short trace cardiotocograph should be carried out to ensure fetal well-being and the uterus should be carefully palpated.

2 The woman should be allowed to walk around or to sit comfortably. She should be re-examined again 4 hours later if the contractions persist.

- If labour has ceased the woman should go home.
- If labour continues and pain relief is required, then it should be given.

• If the cervix continues to efface but not dilate and progress falls more than 2 hours to the right of the partogram (see Fig. 6.2), an attempt should be made to rupture the membranes and labour should be stimulated by Syntocinon.

• In 85% of cases, labour will progress rapidly and will reach a normal active phase.

• In 15% of cases, adequate uterine activity fails to cause cervical dilatation. If, after 4–8 hours of Syntocinon, the cervix is not further dilated, then a Caesarean section should be performed.

PLP is primarily a disease of primigravidae as the multigravidous tend to efface and dilate their cervix at the same time.

Secondary arrest of cervical dilatation

The woman enters the active phase of labour, reaches 5–7 cm dilatation and then the cervix stops dilating (Fig. 6.3). Uterine contractions have become less frequent and may even stop.

• The fetal head engages in the occipitotransverse position and, if it is well flexed and asynclitic, will undergo rotation in the mid-cavity to the direct occipitoanterior position. Poor flexion leads to failure of rotation in the mid-cavity; this leads to persistent occipitotransverse position.

• Syntocinon i.v. leads to regular, coordinated uterine contractions that initially cause the fetal head to flex. In most cases (85%) this allows the head to rotate so that a spontaneous vaginal delivery will occur.

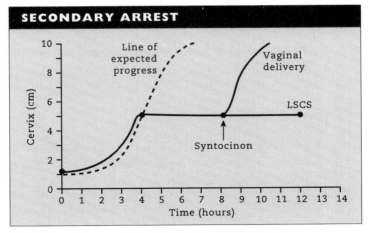

Fig. 6.3 Secondary arrest of cervical dilatation and outcomes.

- If Syntocinon administration over 4 hours (multigravida) or 8 hours (primigravida) fails to lead to further cervical dilatation, a Caesarean section should be carried out for CPD. This occurs in about 15% of cases.
- This is a benign condition as far as the fetus is concerned and very rarely leads to fetal distress.

Primary dysfunctional labour

This is the most worrying of the abnormalities of labour for it can lead to:
- Fetal distress in a well-grown or a large baby.
- Prolonged labour leading to an increase in maternal fear and anxiety.
- Incoordinate uterine activity which increases maternal pain.
- Maternal dehydration which leads to maternal acidosis.

The release of catecholamines stimulates uterine activity to arise from the lower segment. This means that the fundus and the lower uterine segment contract against each other and the cervix fails to dilate or dilates very slowly.

Maternal dehydration and acidosis lead to hydrogen ions competing with calcium (the final common pathway for smooth muscle contraction) and further dysfunctional uterine activity occurs.

Figure 6.4 illustrates a typical case. The causes are:
- A malpresentation such as a brow.
- Occipitoposterior position.
- Relative cephalopelvic disproportion: this means that the fetus is only just small enough to pass through the pelvis but, if all goes well, it will succeed. If there is poor flexion or rotation, delay occurs.

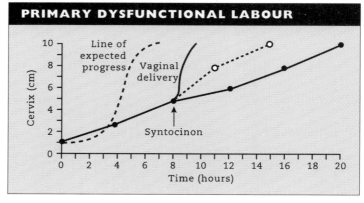

Fig. 6.4 Primary dysfunctional labour.

Once diagnosed, the dysfunction is treated with Syntocinon. In very few cases the rate of cervical dilatation returns to normal, but often the rate of dilatation can be increased. The outcome is:

- Spontaneous vaginal delivery (15%).
- Caesarean section for fetal distress (50%).
- An instrumental delivery (35%). Care should be taken because, even if full dilatation of the cervix is obtained, the fetus may still be high in mid-cavity. This could lead to a difficult, rotation forceps delivery.

Cephalopelvic disproportion

Classically, cephalopelvic disproportion (CPD) is classified as follows:

1   *Absolute*. There is no possibility of a normal vaginal delivery even if the mechanisms of labour are completely correct. In the western world, this condition is extremely rare; it may be due to the following:

- Fetal hydrocephalus.
- Congenitally abnormal pelvis such as Robert's or Naegele's pelvis in which one or both sacral ala are missing leading to a narrowing of the pelvic inlet.
- A pelvis that has been damaged usually due to a severe roll-over road traffic accident in youth.
- A pelvis that has been grossly distorted from osteomalacia.

2   *Relative CPD*. This means that the baby is large but would pass through the pelvis if the mechanisms of labour function correctly. If, however, the head is deflexed or fails to rotate in the mid-cavity then prolonged, abnormal labour will occur.

The above definitions do not include estimates of the weight of the baby or X-ray measurements of the pelvis. CPD can only truly be diag-nosed after a trial of labour. This means awaiting the onset of spontaneous labour and, if that labour becomes prolonged and abnormal, stimulating with Syntocinon as described above.

CPD may be suspected antenatally from women who are less than 5′2″ (1.58 m) in height. These women tend to have a small gynaecoid pelvis but they usually have small babies. In a cephalic presentation there is now little evidence that X-ray pelvimetry or a CT scan helps in management. These women should have a trial of labour and in many cases will deliver vaginally.

All women with a high head at term should have an obvious cause excluded by an ultrasound examination. This will diagnose placenta prae-via, uterine fibroids, or an ovarian cyst as the cause. In the absence of these findings, one should suspect that the cause is CPD.

Head fitting tests and X-ray pelvimetry have only a small role in the management of women with a cephalic presentation because the correct management is the proper use of a trial of labour.

Trial of labour

This somewhat old-fashioned term warns the labour ward staff that CPD is suspected. It is normal to wait for spontaneous labour as this is thought to be more efficient than induced labour. The woman is at risk of Caesarean section and therefore should have the following:

- An indwelling i.v. cannula.
- Oral ranitidine.

Labour is managed as usual with Syntocinon being administered if the rate of cervical dilatation falls to the right of the cervical partogram (Fig. 6.5).

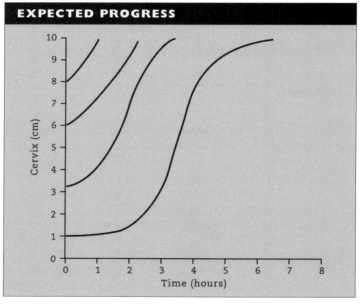

Fig. 6.5 Partograms of expected progress. Start charting at stage of cervix dilatation when woman is admitted.

Malpresentations and malpositions

BREECH PRESENTATION

Incidence
2–3%, commoner in preterm deliveries.

Aetiology
• The ratio of amniotic fluid volume to fetal size may be high, allowing freer movement (e.g. polyhydramnios and before 32 weeks).
• Extended legs of the fetus can splint and prevent flexion of the fetal trunk so stopping further turning and causing the fetus to stay as a breech presentation.
• Fetuses in multiple pregnancies may interfere with each other's movements.
• Something might be filling the lower segment (e.g. placenta praevia or fibroids).
• Fetal malformations may prevent cephalic presentation (e.g. hydrocephaly).

Types (Fig. 6.6)
Flexed or extended knee joints.
1 Fully flexed fetus with both knees flexed: a complete or full breech.
2 Neither knee joint flexed so that both legs are extended: a frank breech or breech with extended legs. This is the commonest presentation.
3 One leg flexed and the other leg extended: an incomplete breech.
4 Both hips extended; a footling. Only occurs with very small babies.

On vaginal examination, the breech presentation in labour is described according to the relation of the fetal sacrum to the maternal pelvis (Fig. 6.7).

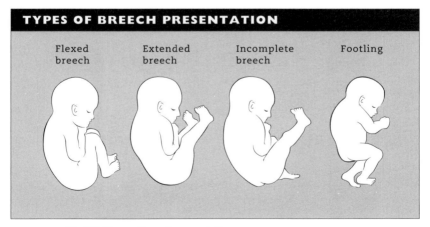

TYPES OF BREECH PRESENTATION

Flexed breech | Extended breech | Incomplete breech | Footling

Fig. 6.6 Types of breech presentation.

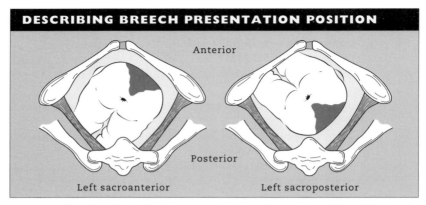

DESCRIBING BREECH PRESENTATION POSITION

Anterior

Posterior

Left sacroanterior   Left sacroposterior

Fig. 6.7 Using the fetal sacrum as the denominator, the position of the breech presentation is described.

Diagnosis

Abdominal examination
No head is felt at the lower end and a hard, rounded knob is ballotable at the upper end of the uterus.

Vaginal examination
Confirms there is no head in the pelvis.

Investigations
Ultrasound scan confirms the situation.

Management of a breech presentation in pregnancy

1   From about 33 weeks onwards external cephalic version (ECV) is worthwhile trying without general anaesthesia, provided it is easy to perform. If the mother is Rh-negative, anti-*D* immunoglobulin should be given after the first attempt.

- Listen to the fetal heart immediately before and after the procedure.
- If it works, the woman should be seen weekly to ensure the fetus stays as a cephalic presentation.
- If it fails, the woman should be asked to come back the following week for another attempt.
- Reasons for failure of ECV:
  - (a) Breech too deeply engaged in pelvis.
  - (b) Too tense a uterus.
  - (c) Too tense an abdominal wall.

(d) Fetal abnormality
(e) Undiagnosed twins   } therefore do an ultrasound.

- Contra-indications to doing ECV.
  (a) Previous uterine scar from Caesarean section.
  (b) Hypertension in the mother.
  (c) Planned delivery by Caesarean section anyway.
  (d) Ruptured membranes.
  (e) Multiple pregnancy.
  (f) Antepartum haemorrhage.

2   If version has not occurred by 36–38 weeks, preparations for breech delivery must take place.

3   A standing lateral X-ray of the pelvis should be done for all primiparous patients and any multiparous women who have delivered a baby of <3.5 kg in the past. In a breech delivery the head (the largest and hardest part of the fetus) is coming last and it is too late to wait and see if this fits the pelvis then.

4   It is wise to deliver most breech presentations by 41 weeks. If the woman has not gone into spontaneous labour before this time then induce or do an elective Caesarean section.

5   If there is any variation from normal, many obstetricians will deliver a breech-presenting baby by elective Caesarean section at 38–39 weeks.

Management of breech presentation in labour

First stage

1   There is an increased risk of early rupture of the membranes; when they do, a vaginal examination should be made to exclude a prolapse of the cord.

2   Uterine action may well be hypotonic and oxytocic drugs may be required to stimulate labour.

3   With increased risk of operative delivery and general anaesthesia, feeding should be kept to a minimum and i.v. fluids given.

4   For the same reasons, an epidural anaesthetic is a good method of pain relief as the delivery can rapidly be changed to an operative delivery if necessary.

Second stage

1   Delivery is by the most senior obstetrician or midwife available with an anaesthetist close to the labour ward in case of sudden need. A paediatrician should be at the delivery.

2   A propped up dorsal position of the mother is the easiest to manage. The labour bed should be capable of breaking in the middle after delivery of the baby's body, so that the mother can assume a lithotomy position.

3   The buttocks progress down the birth canal and, when on the point of crowning, a generous episiotomy is performed.

4   The baby will often progress as far as the umbilicus with the mother's own expulsive efforts. The legs are assisted down, especially if extended.

5   Commonly, the arms are flexed across the chest and so delivery occurs readily with the next contraction.

6   If the arms are extended they have to be manipulated down.

7   After delivery of the body, it is allowed to hang and traction may be gently applied to the legs until the suboccipital region appears under the maternal pubis.

8   The head is delivered with forceps, the blades applied on either side of the fetal cheeks and the body held up by an assistant. This allows controlled traction of the fetal head. The face is delivered over the mother's perineum and the nose and mouth are cleared of mucus and liquor, allowing the baby to breathe. The rest of the head is very slowly delivered, not allowing any sudden decompression to occur for this could result in pressure alterations inside the skull and so venous wall, tears and bleeding.

Other methods of controlled head delivery do exist but these are used only if delivery is by a person unskilled in the use of forceps.

Third stage

1   Syntometrine is given with the delivery of the head for there is an increased risk of PPH.

2   The placenta is delivered as described in normal labour.

Breech extraction

Instead of allowing a natural delivery of the breech, it may have to be accelerated because of:

- Fetal distress.
- Maternal distress.
- Lack of advance in second stage.

These are the same indications for forceps delivery in a cephalic presentation. Breech extraction must only be by senior staff.

Caesarean section

This should be done if vaginal delivery is considered too hazardous because:

- Mild pelvis contraction.

- Fetus thought to be under 1.5 kg (32–34 weeks' gestation).
- Fetus thought to be over 3.5 kg.
- Fetus in unfavourable attitude.
- Multiple pregnancy.
- Other complications, e.g. pre-eclampsia or diabetes.
- Non-descent of buttocks in labour.

Risks to the fetus of breech delivery

Perinatal mortality in all breech deliveries is × 2 or × 3 that of cephalic presentations but this is made up mainly of premature births (26–30 weeks). Mature breech deliveries (36+ weeks) in reputable centres have no higher risk than mature cephalic deliveries. Hence the reasons for mortality are:

- Prematurity.
- Intracranial damage: subdural and intracranial haemorrhage (too rapid delivery of the head).
- Rarely hypoxia. This may be:
    - (a) Before delivery (prolapsed cord).
    - (b) At the time of delivery (too slow delivery of the head).

SHOULDER PRESENTATION (TRANSVERSE LIE)

Incidence
0.3% of all deliveries.

Aetiology
As for other malpresentation but most commonly:
1 Polyhydramnios causing an increased ratio of fluid to fetus.
2 Something preventing the engagement of the head in the pelvis:
   - Placenta praevia.
   - Fibroids.
   - Contracted pelvis.
3 Abnormal shape of uterus (subseptate or arcuate uterus).
4 Second twin.

Diagnosis
1 Abdominal examination—the head is in one flank and the buttocks in the other. Commonly, the fetus can be rotated to a cephalic presentation quite readily but reverts to a transverse position.
2 Vagnial examination—the pelvis is empty of presenting parts.
3 Investigation: ultrasound scan confirms diagnosis.

Management of transverse lie in pregnancy and labour

1   Before 36 weeks, ECV may be attempted and the woman referred back to the following week's clinic, but the position is usually self-curing.

2   Past 37 weeks in a multiparous patient, and after 38 weeks in a nulliparous one, admission to hospital should be advised, where ECV is attempted each day.

3   Should the woman go to term with the fetus still in a transverse position, management may be by either of the following:

  • *A stabilizing induction*: ECV is done in the labour ward. The fetal head is held over the brim of the mother's pelvis and high membrane rupture is performed with a Drew Smythe catheter. Amniotic fluid escapes and the head often sinks into the pelvis. Labour follows in the normal fashion.

  • *An elective Caesarean section*. In the Western world this may be the safer line of treatment for the fetus since it cuts down the risks of prolapsed cord during labour, but it does leave the mother with a scarred uterus for future pregnancies.

4   Occasionally a woman is admitted in mid or late labour with a transverse lie. This would lead to an impacted shoulder presentation, the folded fetus having been driven a varying amount down the pelvis, depending on how far labour has gone. Treatment is by immediate Caesarean section even if the fetus is dead.

OCCIPITOPOSTERIOR POSITIONS

The fetal head usually engages in the pelvic brim in the occipitotransverse position (long axis of head fitting into maximum diameter of bean-shaped pelvic brim). When labour starts, the head is driven down the birth canal and rotates (Fig. 6.8).

1   80% rotate forward through 90° to an occipitoanterior position.

2   15% undergo long internal rotation through 270° to become occipitoanterior having gone through directly occipitoposterior on the way.

3   3% rotate back 90° to a directly occipitoposterior position (this may include some of those in group **2** that never completed the long rotation).

4   2% stay in the transverse and descend in this position. A minority of these might rotate on the perineum but most end up in transverse arrest.

Incidence

Depending on the time in labour when the woman is examined vaginally and on the stage that fetal head rotation has reached, many will be in a transitional occipitoposterior or occipitotransverse position. About half of these will be rotating out of this **2**, another quarter will become

ROTATION OF THE FETAL HEAD

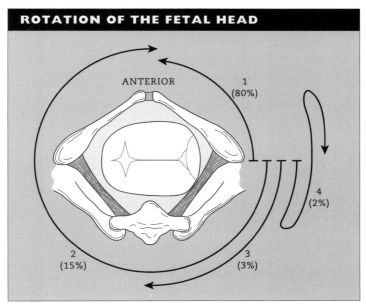

Fig. 6.8 Rotation of the fetal head from the occipitolateral as it descends the birth canal (see text).

directly occipitoposterior **3** and another quarter will remain in the transverse **4**.

Aetiology

Pelvis
Flat sacrum with loss of pelvic curve and room for rotation (Fig. 6.9).

Uterus
Poor or disorganized uterine contractions do not push the fetal head down and so there is no impetus to rotate.

Head
Poor flexion so that larger diameters present (sub-occipitofrontal — 10.5 cm).

Analgesia
Epidural analgesia causes pelvic floor relaxation. This allows the gutter

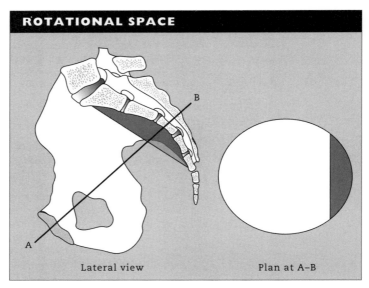

Fig. 6.9 Straight sacrum takes away rotational area from the mid-cavity of the pelvis.

of the levator ani muscles to become lax so not directing the occiput anteriorly. This is associated with lack of fetal head rotation.

Diagnosis

Pregnancy
Occasionally, by abdominal palpation when in a cephalic presentation, the back cannot be felt in the flank but fetal limbs can be felt all over the front of the uterus. The head is often not engaged after the time it would be expected to be.

Labour
• Abdominal palpation as above.
• Vaginal examination feeling the sutures and fontanelles. Both anterior and posterior fontanelle can be felt (deflexion) and the λ-shaped posterior fontanelle is in the anterior quadrant of the pelvis.

Management in pregnancy
Leave alone.

Management in labour
Laissez-faire. Await events for many will rotate spontaneously. Prepare for a longer labour because:

- Pelvis may be minimally contracted or sacrum flattened.
- Incoordinate uterine contractions.
- Deflexed fetal head.

Therefore:

1 Watch progress by both:
- Abdominal assessment of engagement and descent of fetal head.
- Vaginal assessment:
  - (a) Head in relation to ischial spines.
  - (b) Rotation of head.
  - (c) Dilatation of cervix which is often poorly applied to the head.
  - (d) Check no prolapse of cord by vaginal examination straight after membranes rupture.

2 Women often wish to push before the cervix is fully dilated. If the occiput is posterior there is extra pressure on the sacrum and rectum. Frequent vaginal examinations are needed to make accurate assessments of the progress of labour.

3 Watch maternal condition. Especially remember:
- Labour will be long, so maintain morale.
- Pain relief should be thorough—epidural anaesthesia is good in this situation. If such regional anaesthesia is unacceptable to the woman, many would use morphine or diamorphine for this problem.
- No food and little fluids by mouth (general anaesthetic may be wanted). Give i.v. fluids.

4 If head stays directly occipitoposterior, delivery may occur spontaneously but, since larger diameters are passing through birth canal, the mother will have to work harder and a generous episiotomy will be required. Face-to-pubis delivery will occur.

5 If head stays in occipitotransverse, it will not deliver spontaneously. It must be rotated to deliver and this will require good analgesia, maybe epidural or general anaesthesia. Rotation and delivery may be by:
- Manual rotation to the occipitoanterior position and subsequent forceps delivery.
- Kielland's straight forceps rotation and subsequent delivery. These forceps have no pelvic curve.
- Vacuum extraction. This applies only a linear pull on the fetal head so that any rotation can occur as determined by the pelvic muscles and bones.

6 Give i.v. Syntometrine with the crowning of the head for the risks of post-partum haemorrhage are greatly increased. Deliver the placenta promptly after the baby is born.

7 Be prepared to repair the rather large episiotomy quickly.

8 Because of the difficulties inherent in vaginal delivery of a fetus in the occipitoposterior position, many obstetricians will opt for a short trial of uterine contraction (often augmented by i.v. Syntocinon) with a Caesarean section if this policy does not work in 4−6 hours.

Results

Mother
Following the operative delivery and the bigger episiotomy, vaginal and vulval oedema and haematomata are more frequent.

Baby
Because of the longer labour and high incidence of operative delivery, perinatal mortality and morbidity are raised. The increased mortality is due to hypoxia and birth trauma. The morbidity is from these and the results of intracranial haemorrhage.

FACE PRESENTATION

As the fetal head gets driven down the birth canal, the front of the head can become extended (Fig. 6.10). Distinguish from face-to-pubis delivery (p. 177).

Incidence
0.3% of all deliveries.

Aetiology
1   Lax uterus, multiple pregnancy, polyhydramnios.
2   Deflexed fetal head.

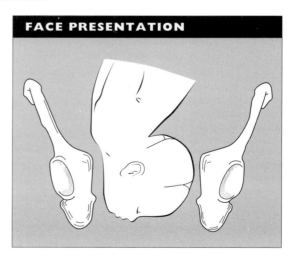

Fig. 6.10 Face presentation. Well engaged in the mentolateral position.

3   Shape of fetal head:
  • Dolichocephalic (long head).
  • Anencephalic (no cranium).

Mechanism

Head descends with face leading. Chin (mentum) used as denominator to determine rotation.

85% engage in the mentotransverse (sub-mentobregmatic diameter—10 cm). With descent, most rotate to mentoanterior on the pelvic floor, the fetal chin coming behind the maternal pubis. After further descent, the chin can escape from under the lower back of pubis and the head is then delivered over the vulva by flexion.

Up to this point, the mechanisms of flexion/extension of the fetal head are the reverse of those with a vertex presentation. After delivery of the head, however, the external rotations are the same allowing the fetal shoulders to negotiate the pelvis.

A few face presentations rotate from the transverse to mentoposterior, so that the fetal chin is in the curve of the mother's sacrum; the fetal occiput and back are crushed into each other behind the public bone. Further descent is unlikely for the head cannot extend further and so cannot negotiate the forward curve of the birth canal. Caesarean section is needed.

Diagnosis

Rarely made before labour and of little significance if it is.

Abdomen
  • Longitudinal lie with body nearer to mid-axis of uterus.
  • More head felt on the same side as back (Fig. 6.11).

Vaginal examination
  • Do not expect the face to feel like the newborn baby's face. Oedema always obscures facial parts.
  • Supraorbital ridges lead to the birdge of the nose.
  • Mouth has hard gums in it and may suck on the examining finger.

Management

In pregnancy
  • Await events.
  • Membranes may rupture early (examine vaginally to exclude prolapsed cord).

WELL FLEXED HEAD AND FACE PRESENTATIONS

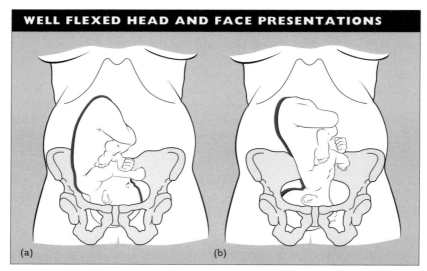

(a)   (b)

Fig. 6.11 On abdominal palpation, with a well-flexed head (a) the fetal back is felt right down to the maternal pelvis brim and most of the head mass is on the opposite side. With a face presentation (b) one loses the back and feels no shoulder. The head mass is on the same side.

- Check that pelvis is adequate and that fetus is not oversized. If either, consider elective Caesarean section for face presentation in labour has a higher risk.
- Check with ultrasound that the fetus is not an anencephalic for this might alter management.

In labour
- If anterior rotation to mentoanterior, a longer labour but spontaneous delivery will probably occur (90%).
- If head stays in mentotransverse, either manual rotation to mentoanterior and forceps extraction, or Kielland's forceps rotation and extraction.
- If face rotates posteriorly, this is impossible to deliver vaginally. Hence, deliver by Caesarean section.

Results

Mother
Higher morbidity associated with operative delivery.

Baby

Higher mortality:

- Abnormalities incompatible with life (anencephaly).
- In the normal, hypoxia and cerebral congestion.

BROW PRESENTATION

A very poorly flexed head may present the largest diameter of the skull: mentovertex (13 cm) (Fig. 6.12).

Incidence
0.1% of all deliveries.

Diagnosis
Rarely made before labour and of little significance if it is.

Abdomen

- Head feels big.
- Not well engaged.
- Groove between occiput and back. Head felt on both sides of fetus (Fig. 6.13).

Vaginal examination

- Anterior fontanelle presents.
- Supra-orbital ridges and base of nose can be felt at edge of field.

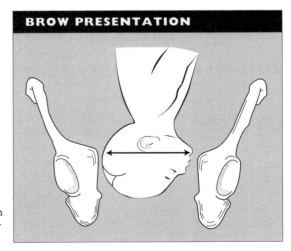

BROW PRESENTATION

Fig. 6.12 Brow presentation with mentovertex diameter presenting.

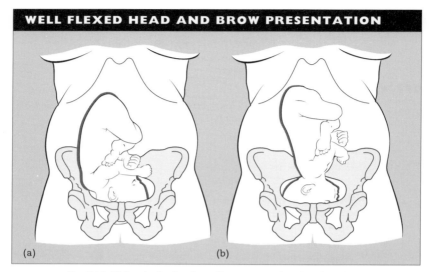

Fig. 6.13 Abdominal palpation of brow presention showing (a) a well-flexed head and (b) a poorly flexed head.

Management

In pregnancy
• Await events. No point in trying to convert to more favourable presentation.
• Membranes may rupture early (examine vaginally to exclude prolapsed cord).

In labour
• If diagnosed early, await events for some convert spontaneously to face (by further extension) or vertex (by flexion).
• If presentation persists, it will be impossible to deliver vaginally. Hence deliver by Caesarean section.
• If fetus is dead or there is gross hydrocephaly, the destructive operation of perforation of head and vaginal extraction is possible provided the operator is skilled in these arts but in the western world these are a diminishing number.

Results

Mother
Higher morbidity associated with operative delivery.

Baby
Because of wider use of Caesarean section, morbidity and mortality rates are low.

Induction of labour

Definition
A planned initiation of labour.

Incidence
Varies with the population and the type of obstetric cases seen; in the UK between 5% and 25%.

Indications
1   Maternal disease:
   - Existing before pregnancy, e.g. diabetes.
   - Occurring in pregnancy, e.g. pre-eclampsia.
2   Fetal disease, e.g. Rh disease.
3   Fetuses at risk from reduced placental perfusion, showing SGA.
   In the UK the most common indications are:
   - Post-maturity (or more strictly post-dates).
   - SGA.
   - Maternal disease.
   - Rh incompatibility.
   - Fetal death or abnormality.

In addition, there are several softer indications which obstetricians commonly employ for which there is little or no scientific basis. These are:
   - Poor past obstetric history.
   - A pregnancy resulting from infertility treatment.
   - Recurrent unexplained APH.
   - For the woman or her partner's convenience.

The commonest means of induction of labour in the UK is a combination of medical and surgical means. The usual system is:

1   Give prostaglandin in either vaginal pessaries (E_2, 2 mg) or as a gel (1 or 2 mg E_2). In up to 40%, this will start labour on its own and no further action is required.
2   If not, 4 hours later, repeat the PG and wait 1 hour.
3   If no action after an hour, rupture membranes.
4   Administer Syntocinon if uterine contractions do not follow closely or if labour becomes prolonged and abnormal so that the rate of cervical dilatation is to the right of the cervical partogram.

Prostaglandins

A ubiquitous group of fatty acids found in many body fluids first described in seminal plasma, hence their name. Prostaglandins E and F stimulate uterine activity and are involved in the initiation of normal labour.

Mode of action

This is directly on the muscle cells. A secondary effect is that a uterus primed with prostaglandins will respond much better to i.v. Syntocinon.

Route

1   *Intravenous.* May have side-effects of diarrhoea, vomiting and gastro-intestinal colic; this route has been abandoned for labour induction.

2   *Intramuscular.* This route has never really been used to stimulate labour but direct intramyometrium injections of prostaglandins can be life-saving if the woman has a torrential, atonic PPH.

3   *The oral route.* This is not commonly used because of the side-effects of gastrointestinal colic and diarrhoea.

4   *Extra-amniotic.* A fine catheter passed through the cervix comes to lie between the membranes and the uterine side-wall. Prostaglandins are then injected through the catheter. It is an unnecessarily complicated pro-cedure; in some cases the membranes rupture. This method has been abandoned in most units.

5   *Intra-amniotic.* By direct injection of prostaglandin into the amniotic sac; may be used to induce therapeutic abortion but is not used to induce labour.

6   *Intravaginal.* Putting either a gel or a pessary into the vagina.

Uses

1   *To cause cervical ripening.* If the cervix is long and closed it may be ripened by a 2-mg prostaglandin pessary. This has the risk that some of these women will go into labour and in such cases, particularly if the ripening is taking place overnight, the fetus may be unmonitored.

2   *To induce labour.* A dose of PGE_2 in a 2 mg pessary or a 1 or 2 mg gel I placed high in the vagina. If labour is not established and the cervix is not dilating some 3–4 hours later, then the PGE_2 may be repeated. Four hours after this it is usual to do an artificial rupture of membranes (ARM) and then to add Syntocinon if necessary.

Syntocinon

This is an artificially produced oxytocic agent which mimics the activity of the normally released oxytocin. In normal labour, oxytocin is not detectable until the cervix has reached 7 cm dilatation.

Nowadays labour is not commonly induced with oxytocin alone; it is used:

• When prostaglandin pessaries and ARM fail to result in uterine activity and active dilatation of the cervix.

• To augment abnormal labour when the rate of cervical dilatation has fallen to the right of the cervical partogram.

ARTIFICIAL RUPTURE OF MEMBRANES

Figure 6.14 illustrates rupture of the forewaters in order to induce or accelerate labour. This is carried out with an amnihook or by a pair of Kocher's forceps.

The following conditions should exist before ARM is carried out:

• The fetal head or presenting part should be firmly engaged.

• The woman should be informed of the procedure and the reasons for it; oral consent should be obtained.

SUCCESS OF INDUCTION OF LABOUR

Even with an unfavourable cervix the use of prostaglandins, ARM and Syntocinon should result in a failed induction rate of no more than 5%.

Management of women who have a failed induction depends upon the obstetrician's opinion, which may be either of the following:

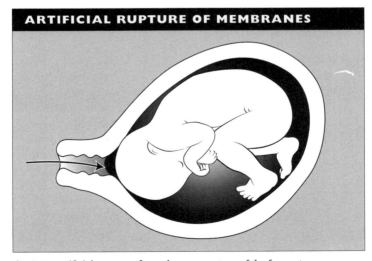

Fig. 6.14 Artificial rupture of membranes: rupture of the forewaters (arrowed).

1   The need for induction indicated a need for delivery and therefore failure of induction should lead to a Caesarean section.

2   The indications for induction were borderline and it is therefore reasonable to stop the induction process and attempt it again the next day. This can only be carried out if the membranes have not been ruptured. It is not to be encouraged as it leads to the woman's loss of confidence in the method.

The state of the cervix

Table 6.1 illustrates the Bishop's score; a weighted means of assessing how likely it is that the woman will go into labour. Women with a Bishop's score of >6 are considered favourable and failed induction rates are usually less than 1%.

Risks of induction

• Uterine hyperstimulation may lead to fetal distress and so to a Caesarean section.

• Prolonged rupture of the membranes may increase the risk of intrauterine infection.

• Prolonged labour may lead to a Caesarean section.

• Women whose labours are induced have a higher incidence of Caesarean section (a risk factor ×3). Often this is due to the reason for the induction, e.g. an SGA fetus, but in many cases it is due to prolonged labour.

• Nowadays, with widespread ultrasound examinations in early pregnancy for dating, it is rare to induce a patient and find an unexpectedly preterm baby, but this can happen.

THE BISHOP'S SCORE			
Cervix	**0**	**1**	**2**
Dilatation (cm)	0	1–2	3–4
Consistency	Firm	Medium	Soft
Length (cm)	>2	1–2	<1
Position	Posterior	Mid	Anterior
Station of head above ischial spines (cm)	3	2	1

Table 6.1 The Bishop's score.

• Precipitate labour. Women who have had several children already should be induced carefully for prostaglandins may lead to delivery within 1 or 2 hours and this may cause cerebral damage to the baby.

Preterm labour

Definition
Labour occurring at <37 completed weeks' gestation.

Incidence
6% of deliveries occur before 37 weeks' gestation.
2% of deliveries occur before 34 weeks' gestation.

Prognosis
This depends upon:
• The availability of a neonatal intensive care unit. All infants born at <30 weeks' gestation should be transferred to a hospital that contains a neonatal intensive care unit if time and maternal/fetal condition allow.
• The gestational age and birth weight. The perinatal team at a typical obstetric and paediatric combined unit usually achieves a 50% survival rate at 26 weeks of gestation.
• The condition of the baby at birth. Asphyxiated infants are more likely to die later from RDS.
• Immediate neonatal management. Figure 6.15 illustrates the avoidable factors that worsen surfactant deficiency and subsequent RDS.
• The use of steroids to improve the maturity of the fetal lungs in fetuses of less than 34 weeks' gestation.

Diagnosis
Half the women who present with painful contractions before 37 weeks' gestation will stop spontaneously. Conversely preterm labour may be insidious. The following plan is therefore recommended:
1   Look for a cause for preterm labour (Box 6.1).
2   If membranes are intact, a vaginal examination should be performed.
3   The fetal heart rate and uterine activity should be electronically recorded continuously.
4   Repeat the vaginal examination 2 hours later if there are more than two contractions every 10 min. Change in cervical effacement or dilatation confirms preterm labour.
5   Check fibronectin levels in cervical fluid, elevation may indicate imminent labour.

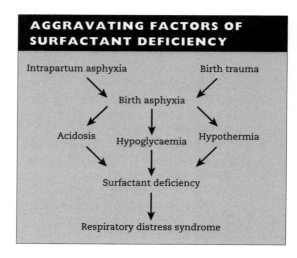

Fig. 6.15 Avoidable perinatal factors that aggravate surfactant deficiency.

CAUSES OF PRETERM LABOUR

Preterm premature rupture of the membranes
Cervical incompetence
Multiple pregnancy
Polyhydramnios
Antepartum haemorrhage
Fetal death
Maternal pyrexia
Uterine abnormalities

Box 6.1 Causes of preterm labour.

Principles of management of ongoing labour (intact membranes)

1 Full electronic monitoring is mandatory.

2 Arrange *in utero* transfer if neonatal intensive care facilities are unavailable.

3 Give tocolytics for 72 hours to allow steroid therapy to mature fetal lungs.

4 If labour is or becomes established epidural analgesia is best.

5 Breech presentations at less than 34 weeks' gestation should probably be delivered by Caesarean section.

Tocolysis

There is no convincing statistical evidence that tocolytic agents usefully prolong pregnancy. However, at <4 cm dilatation they may delay delivery for 72 hours in order to allow time for steroids to act or for the woman to be transferred to a delivery site with an intensive neonatal unit.

Contra-indications

Absolute
- Thyroid disease.
- Cardiac disease.
- Severe hypertension (>160/110 mmHg).
- Sickle cell disease.
- Chorioamnionitis.
- Intrauterine death.

Relative
- Advanced labour, more than 4 cm cervical dilatation.
- APH.
- Maternal diabetes mellitis.

Steroid therapy

Steroids have been shown statistically to reduce the incidence of deaths from RDS between the gestations of 26 and 34 weeks.

Contra-indications
- Evidence of chorioamnionitis.
- Severe hypertension.
- Maternal cardiac disease.
- Asymmetrical growth retardation.

Conduct of a preterm delivery
- The fetal heart should be electronically monitored.
- A senior obstetrician should be present.
- A neonatal paediatrician should be present.
- An elective episiotomy is usually advised.

Preterm premature rupture of membranes (PROM)

PROM refers to rupture of the membranes before the onset of labour. At less than 37 weeks' gestation this is referred to as preterm premature rupture of the membranes (PPROM).

Problems

Risks of preterm delivery versus risk of intrauterine infection.

Confirm the diagnosis
- Avoid vaginal digital examinations.
- Perform a sterile speculum examination.
- If amniotic fluid is seen coming through the cervix, membranes have ruptured.
- The smell of amniotic fluid is characteristic.
- A positive Nitrazine stick test (pH change) is of imprecise help.

Management

PPROM after 34 weeks' gestation
Management is controversial and follows one of two lines:
- Immediate delivery to avoid intrauterine infection. Perinatal mortality because of immaturity is almost identical to that at term. However these babies do have an increased morbidity.
- Perform an amniocentesis to exclude an infection and if not present then manage the woman conservatively.

PPROM at less than 34 weeks' gestation
Care must be individualized but the following lines of management are reasonable:
- *In utero* transfer to a hospital with a neonatal intensive care unit for all women <34 weeks' gestation.
- Perform an amniocentesis. If the amniotic fluid shows organisms, this suggests intrauterine infection and the woman should be delivered.
- Conservative management in the absence of an amniocentesis. In this case, women are delivered for the following reasons:
  (a) Evidence of chorioamnionitis.
  (b) Maturity.
  (c) Spontaneous onset of labour.

Chorioamnionitis
This is usually diagnosed by one or more of the following:
- Maternal temperature and tachycardia.
- Tender uterus.
- A foul-smelling vaginal discharge.
- Fetal tachycardia.
- Rise in maternal white cell count.
- Organisms in amniotic fluid.

Management
I   Obtain high vaginal swab, a MSU and blood culture.

2   Induce labour. Caesarean section is preferably avoided because of the risk of maternal infection but it is indicated in the following circumstances:
- Fetal distress.
- Preterm breech or other abnormal lie.
- A failed induction.

3   The current philosophy is to withhold antibiotics until after delivery.

Then start i.v. broad-spectrum antibiotics such as cephradine and metronidazole for both mother and baby. These ideas may change.

Presentation and prolapse of the cord

PRESENTATION OF THE CORD

During labour, loops of cord may be felt ahead of the presenting part; if the membranes are intact this is not dangerous. The cord will probably slip to one side when the presenting part comes down. However, if, in a live fetus, cord presentation is felt at a time of proposed artificial rupture of the membranes, that procedure is better postponed for an hour or so.

PROLAPSE OF THE CORD

If the membranes rupture and the presenting part does not fit the pelvis well, the umbilical cord can be carried through the cervix by the flow of amniotic fluid.

Associated factors

Badly fitting presenting part:
- Occipitoposterior position.
- Breech.
- Face and brow presentations.
- Transverse lie.
- High head:
    - (a)   Preterm delivery.
    - (b)   Small baby.
    - (c)   Multiparity.

Incidence

1 : 300 of all deliveries.

Findings

Loops of cord may:
- Pass through cervix and stay in vagina.
- Pass out of vulva.

Dangers

Fetus is put at risk of cutting off blood supply.
- Spasm of umbilical arteries from:
    - (a) Cooling.
    - (b) Drying.
    - (c) Altered pH.
    - (d) Handling.
- Mechanical compression between presenting part and maternal bony pelvis.

Diagnosis

1   The fetal heart may show a sudden alteration in rate or rhythm soon after membrane rupture.

2   Loops of cord appear at the vulva or are felt in the vagina at examination. Do *not* handle cord too much. Just determine if the vessels are pulsating.

Management

If fetus mature and alive

1   Deliver immediately:
- If cervix <9 cm dilated—Caesarean section.
- If cervix >9 cm and favourable cephalic presentation in a multiparous patient—vacuum extraction.
- If cervix fully dilated—forceps or breech extraction.

2   If immediate delivery impossible (e.g. prolapsed cord occurs outside a properly equipped obstetrical unit):
- Keep cord moist, warm and do not handle. If outside vulva, return cord to vagina.
- Prevent compression of cord between the presenting part and the bony pelvis: put mother in lateral position with pelvis raised on pillows; press up presenting part with the fingers in the vagina.

Keep these precautions until delivery about to occur, i.e. if the mother must travel in an ambulance, the doctor or midwife goes with her still doing a vaginal examination to continue to hold up presenting part.

Do not waste time trying to put the cord back into the uterus above the presenting part. Each attempt may allow more loops to come down and the additional handling increases spasm.

If fetus dead

There is no urgency for there is no increased risk to the mother. Allow events to proceed; the cord will not obstruct labour.

Prognosis

Maternal
Increased morbidity risks of operative delivery.

Fetal
Depends where the woman is when the prolapse occurs and at what stage of labour. If the mother is in hospital and the prolapse is in the second stage, the fetal loss is <3%. Should she be at home with a first stage prolapse, figures as high as 70% loss occur.

Postpartum haemorrhage (PPH)

Bleeding from the genital tract after delivery of the fetus.

PRIMARY PPH

Definition
A blood loss in excess of 500 ml from the vagina within 24 hours of birth.

Incidence
Varies with use of oxytocic drugs. From 1% to 8% of all deliveries.

Causes
1   Uterus does not contract and so prevent bleeding from placental site. Haemostasis is mostly mechanical immediately after delivery, with muscle fibres kinking blood vessels (Fig. 6.16).
2   Partly separated placenta — uterus cannot contract properly and so placental bed bleeds.
3   Retention of separated placenta — lower areas of the uterus contract so that the placenta is trapped and cannot be expelled.
4   Tears of the uterus, cervix, vagina or perineum.
5   A clotting defect of blood.

Predisposing factors
- Overstretch of uterus — twins, polyhydramnios.
- Long labour.
- Deep anaesthesia or use of halothane.
- Previous scar on uterus.
- Morbid penetration of placenta.
- Cervical contraction after oxytocic drugs.
- Cornual pockets (Fig. 6.17).

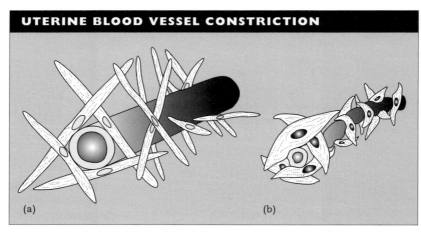

Fig. 6.16 Uterine blood vessels become constricted when the surrounding muscle fibres contract.

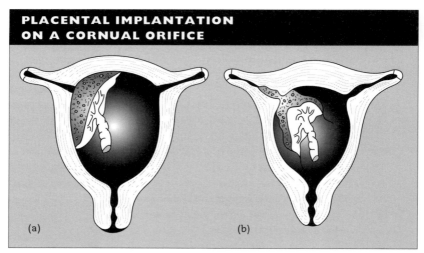

Fig. 6.17 (a) The placenta may implant by chance on a cornual orifice. (b) If the myometrium is hypertrophic in this region, when the uterine muscle contracts after delivery, a part of the placenta may be trapped in a cornual pocket or diverticulum.

- Vaginal operative delivery, especially if cervix not fully dilated.
- Hypofibrinogenaemia after abruptio placentae.
- Disseminated intravascular coagulopathy.

Diagnosis

Since the definition of a PPH is a loss over 500 ml, an attempt should be made to measure blood loss at delivery. This is rarely accurate since:

1 Not all blood lost is collected:
  - Some on sheets and floor.
  - Some still inside uterus (but lost from intravascular space).
2 Other fluids often included accidentally:
  - Urine.
  - Amniotic fluid.
  - Cleaning-up solutions.

Estimates are made and these are usually smaller in volume than the actual loss, sometimes as much as 50%. Therefore, give treatment on lower estimates of blood loss than would be done at a surgical operation.

Treatment

Prevention

Give oxytocic drug with delivery of baby, e.g. Syntometrine (ergometrine 0.5 mg and oxytocin 5 i.u.) i.m. This is the best way to prevent PPH. There may be an increased risk of retained placenta but that does not kill; PPH does.

Curative

1 Give another dose of oxytocic (possibly ergometrine 0.5 mg i.v.).
2 Have blood taken for crossmatching and put up i.v. drip of Hartmann's solution.
3 Give blood if loss over 1000 ml or woman was anaemic in pregnancy.
4 Determine cause:
  - If placenta out—examine for completeness.
  - If placenta not delivered—make arrangements for removal.

Uterine atony
1 Massage uterus to stimulate contraction.
2 Syntocinon i.v. by continuous drip (10 i.u./500 ml fluid).
3 Bimanually compress uterus (Fig. 6.18).
4 Injection of prostaglandin $PGE_{2\alpha}$ or carboprost directly into uterus.
5 Hysterectomy.

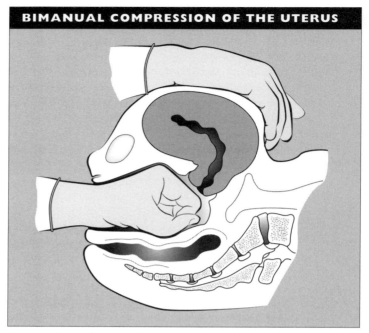

BIMANUAL COMPRESSION OF THE UTERUS

Fig. 6.18 Bimanual compression of the uterus, wrapping it onto the clenched fist in the vagina.

Since the wider use of oxytocics both in prevention and treatment, the last three methods are rarely used and **5** is exceedingly unusual.

Partly separated retained placenta
1   Uterus is often well contracted.
2   Try controlled cord traction again, being careful not to snap cord.
3   Put up i.v. drip with Hartmann's solution while awaiting blood. Give blood if more than 1000 ml loss or patient was anaemic in pregnancy.
4   If placenta still undelivered 20 minutes after birth of the baby, prepare for manual removal. Try one gentle, sterile vaginal examination; placenta may be trapped by the closing cervix and an edge can sometimes be hooked down and the placenta gently eased out.
5   If an epidural is already acting, use this, otherwise a general anaesthetic is needed.
   • Try once more to remove placenta by controlled cord traction just before the anaesthetist induces sleep. Sometimes separation has occurred in the meantime.

- Empty patient's bladder with catheter.
- Cover exploring hand and wrist with antiseptic cream.
- Slip hand through cervix (dilating it slightly if necessary by making a cone of the fingers).
- Follow up cord and separate placenta from uterine wall with fingers.
- Use the hand on the abdominal wall to manipulate the uterus onto the working hand inside the cavity.
- When placenta separated, remove by traction and check it is complete.
- Explore cavity of uterus with fingers for any fragments left behind.
- Give a Syntocinon infusion and prophylactic antibiotics afterwards.

6 If retention of the placenta occurs without a postpartum haemorrhage, the same procedures are done.

7 Very rarely, the placenta may be abnormally adherent:

- Placenta accreta—villi just penetrate into myometrium.
- Placenta increta—villi penetrate deeply into myometrium.
- Placenta percreta—villi penetrate to peritoneum.

Usually this is not possible to diagnose prospectively. If no plane of separation exists (and often there is little bleeding at the time) placenta accreta, increta or percreta must be thought of. Should the patient wish no more children, the safest treatment is hysterectomy. If this is not possible, piecemeal removal is very dangerous and it is better to leave the placenta to atrophy with antibiotic control of infection.

Note: This is a very rare diagnosis made less often as the observer becomes more experienced.

Tears of genital tract

Heavy bleeding may occur from a tear of the cervix despite a well-contracted uterus and a completely expelled placenta.

1 It is difficult to diagnose certainly and requires:

- Adequate general anaesthesia, unless epidural already acting.
- The woman in lithotomy position on a firm bed.
- Good lights and good assistance.
- Several ring forceps and retractors (the vagina and cervix are soft just after delivery and tissues flop into the line of sight).

2 Search cervix systematically using three pairs of ring forceps. If there is a tear:

- Check it does not run up into uterus, especially if at 3 or 9 o'clock.
- Suture with polyglycol absorbable material.

3 Check lower uterine segment with fingers through the cervix. If a tear is found: either repair through abdominal incision or perform a hysterectomy.

4   Check top end of episiotomy or tear which may go into posterior or lateral fornix.
- Repair systematically.

5   Check no actively bleeding vessels in episiotomy or tear.
- Tie them off separately.

Blood clotting defect

(For haematological details see p. 89.)

1   Check that blood taken from an arm vein clots and stays clotted.

2   Check:
- Platelets.
- Coagulation studies.

3   Treat appropriately by fresh blood transfusion:
- Fibrinogen.

4   Remember such a state can allow secondary atony of the myometrium, so watch for that too as a cause of bleeding.

Effects of primary PPH

Rapid loss leads to hypovolaemic shock. If not corrected, this can cause:

1   Death — about 8% of direct maternal deaths follow PPH; half of these are avoidable.

2   Renal shutdown and consequent anuria.

3   Damage to pituitary portal circulation causing necrosis and subsequent Sheehan's syndrome.

4   Postpartum anaemia and chronic ill health.

SECONDARY PPH

This is abnormal vaginal bleeding that occurs after 24 hours following delivery. There is no volumetric definition, women usually present:
- With the passage of clots.
- At 7–10 days with a resumption of fresh vaginal bleeding.

Causes
- Retained pieces of placenta.
- Retained pieces of membrane.
- Retained blood clot.
- Infection of the residual decidua.

Clinical findings
- Fresh red vaginal bleeding and clots.
- A large uterus.
- A tender uterus.
- An open cervical internal os.

Risks
- Substantial bleeding.
- Infection:
    (a) Toxaemia.
    (b) Blocked fallopian tubes.

Treatment
- Admit to hospital.
- Carry out an evacuation of retained products of conception. This should be performed gently by a senior obstetrician because of the risk of perforation of the very soft uterus.
- Give i.v. broad-spectrum antibiotic cover, starting about 1 hour pre-operatively and continuing for a minimum of 5 days. This combats the bacteraemia that may occur and also reduces the risk of subsequent tubal damage.

MASSIVE BLOOD LOSS
Rarely, a haemorrhage of 2–3 litres occurs suddenly at delivery. The woman's life will depend on a well-drilled team having a laid-down policy.

Management
Massive loss from the woman's circulating blood volume of 2–3 litres in a few minutes. For practical purposes consider it has happened if the woman has required more than 2 units of blood quickly.

In anticipation of blood loss all women are routinely grouped and screened for antibodies in the antenatal clinics. Furthermore all at high risk of haemorrhage during labour should be crossmatched prospectively.

Action
1 Put in two large-bore (at least 16 gauge) i.v. cannulae.
2 Contact the duty obstetric registrar, if not already present, and the duty anaesthetic registrar. Call the obstetric consultant.
3 Use one or more of the following fluids.
- Up to 2 litres of Hartmann's solution.
- Up to 1.5 litres of Gelfusin.
- Uncrossmatched blood of the woman's group.
- Crossmatched blood as soon as available.
- Give O Rh-negative blood only as a last resort.
- In an emergency situation the use of blood filters and blood warming devices is not recommended. Pressurized infusion bags should be used.

• Stored blood becomes deficient in platelets and clotting factors. Give 1 unit of fresh frozen plasma (FFP) for every 6 units of blood. The haematologist will advise on platelet replacement.

• If blood sucked out of the peritoneal cavity directly is collected into a sterile, heparinized container it can later be put through *cell sorter* and the cells returned to the woman.

4 Stop the bleeding. If the bleeding is from the uterus:

• Give 0.5 mg of ergometrine i.v. and set up 40 units of Syntocinon in 1 litre of Hartmann's solution to run at 40 drops/minute.

• Commence bimanual compression of the uterus. If trauma, repair uterus.

5 Contact the blood bank. Send at least 20 ml of blood for further crossmatching. Ask for at least 6 units of crossmatched blood.

6 Inform the duty haematologist of the clinical situation, the rate of blood loss and the clotting problems.

7 Insert a central venous line to monitor fluid replacement.

8 One person should be assigned to record-keeping and should record the following:

• Pulse.
• Blood pressure.
• Maternal heart rate, preferably from an ECG.
• Central venous pressure.
• Urine output.
• Amount and type of fluids the woman is given.
• Drugs the woman has received.

9 Prepare for theatre as appropriate.

10 Before proceeding to hysterectomy, the following should be considered:

(a) Direct i.m. injection of 0.5 mg of PGE_2 into the exposed uterus.

(b) Open the broad ligament and ligate the uterine artery on each side.

(c) Ligate internal iliac arteries.

Operative delivery

FORCEPS

The function of which is to get purchase on a rounded object (the fetal head) and to apply traction. This is usually needed to hasten delivery, but it can control the speed of descent, e.g. the aftercoming head in breech delivery.

Usage

Depends on availability of obstetricians. In UK 5–15% of all deliveries.

Mechanism

There are many types of forceps. Basically all have:
- Curved blades to fit around the head (Fig. 6.19).
- Handles to apply traction (Fig. 6.20).

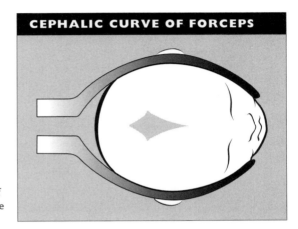

Fig. 6.19 Cephalic curve of a pair of forceps to embrace a fetal head.

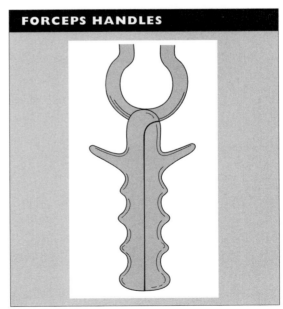

Fig. 6.20 Handles of a pair of forceps to allow traction.

Some have also:

1 A curve in the handle to allow for the curve of the pelvis (Fig. 6.21).

2 If they do not have a pelvic curve, they may be straight-handled to allow rotation manoeuvres (Fig. 6.22).

3 Some have a sliding lock to allow for an asymmetrically aligned head.

Thus there are two basic types. All have curved blades and handles for traction. In addition:

- Traction forceps incorporate **1**.
- Rotation and traction forceps incorporate **1**, **2** and usually **3**.

Indications for use

1 Poor progress in the second stage. No exact time-limits but most would consider the longer limits as 2 hours in a primigravida and half that in a multigravida. If an epidural anaesthetic is being used, these time-limits are usually increased.

2 Clinical fetal distress.
  - Alterations of fetal heart rate and rhythm.
  - Passage of meconium.

3 Biophysical or biochemical signs of fetal hypoxia.
  - On the fetal heart rate trace:
    (a) Tachycardia or bradycardia.

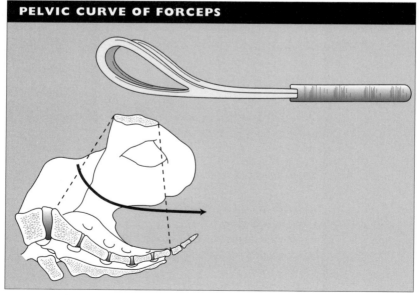

PELVIC CURVE OF FORCEPS

Fig. 6.21 The pelvic curve of the forceps to fit the curved line of advance of a fetus through the pelvis.

DIFFERENCES IN PELVIC CURVES OF FORCEPS

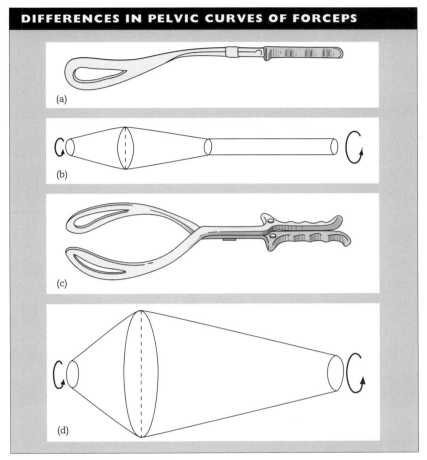

Fig. 6.22 Straight-handled forceps (a) allow rotation to occur in their longitudinal plane so that the cone, subtended by the forceps, (b) is no larger than that made by the head. A pair of forceps with a pelvic curve (c) undergoing the same rotation (d) would make a larger arc and might damage maternal tissues, e.g. bladder and rectum.

    (b) Loss of baseline variability.

    (c) Late decelerations.

    • On fetal blood sampling, scalp capillary blood: base deficit greater than 10 mEq/l; pH below 7.15 in second stage.

4   Maternal distress.

    • A tired woman after a long first stage.

    • One who is frightened or has not had proper analgesia.

5   To prevent fetal morbidity.

- Very immature babies.
- Delivering the head of a breech presentation.

6 To prevent maternal morbidity.
- Women with cardiac or respiratory disease.
- Following a dural tap at attempted epidural injection.

Provisions before use

1 Cervix must be fully dilated.

2 Bladder and rectum should be empty.

3 The membranes must be ruptured.

4 There should be no obvious bar to delivery, e.g. no expected disproportion.

5 Some form of anaesthesia should be used: epidural (if already running), pudendal block or a field block depending on level of presenting part and need for rotation.

6 The woman's legs should be supported in lithotomy position.

7 Full aseptic technique.

8 An episiotomy is nearly always required.

Method

These methods are best learned by watching and helping in the labour ward. Here essentials only are given.

Traction forceps

1 Check the list of provisions before use.

2 Check the head is either occipitoanterior or directly occipitoposterior.

3 Check the forceps blades are a pair and lubricate blades with antiseptic cream.

4 Slip two fingers of right hand up alongside fetal head and hold vaginal tissues back. Make sure no rim of cervix remains.

5 Slide the left blade of the forceps up the palmar aspect of the fingers. Remember the pelvic curve and so start with the handle vertically up (almost over the maternal pubis).

6 Bring handle right down to the fourchette and the blade will now be cupping the parietal eminence of the fetal head.

7 Slip fingers of left hand along other side of fetal head and guide the forceps right blade in.

8 Lock the blades and see they come comfortably together. If they do not, consider the application to be incorrect. Remove blades and start again.

9 Episiotomy as head crowns.

10   Traction so that pull on the head is in line with the relevant part of the birth canal (Fig. 6.23).

Rotation and traction forceps

1   Check the list of provisions before use.

2   Check where the occiput is (usually lateral if rotation is to be employed).

3   Hold forceps with indicator knobs (Fig. 6.24) towards the occiput.

4   Take anterior blade. Slip it over the fetal face and then rotate it through 90° so that it cups the parietal eminence.

5   Apply posterior blade directly with the guiding fingers well up the vagina to protect soft tissues from inclusion in the blade's grip.

6   Lock — often there is asymmetry in the longitudinal plane implying lateral rotation of the head (asynclitism).

7   Keep a thumb between the handles to prevent fetal head compression.

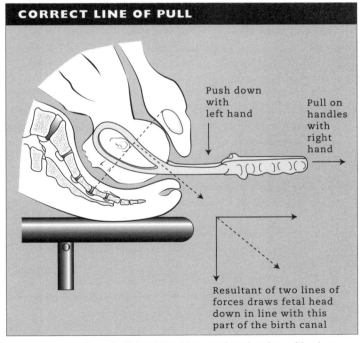

CORRECT LINE OF PULL

Push down with left hand

Pull on handles with right hand

Resultant of two lines of forces draws fetal head down in line with this part of the birth canal

Fig. 6.23 Correct line of pull is achieved by use of two hands working in co-operation, thus performing the task more simply than a pair of axis traction forceps.

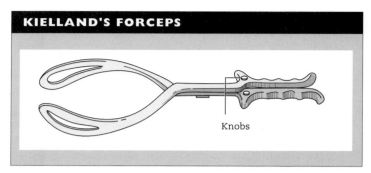

KIELLAND'S FORCEPS

Knobs

Fig. 6.24 Kielland's forceps showing indicator knobs on posterior surface of handles.

8 Gently correct asynclitism while rotating and applying traction. Usually all three movements go together.

9 Traction so that the pull at the level of the head is in line with the birth canal.

Forceps to the head of a breech presentation

1 Check there is no gross disproportion.

2 Have fetal body held up by assistant.

3 Slip blades one at a time over the fetal cheeks so that they cup the parietal eminence (similar to cephalic presentations but 180° opposite).

4 Deliver face over perineum—episiotomy has been done earlier.

5 As soon as nose and mouth delivered, have the upper respiratory passages cleared by mucus aspiration.

6 Slow down delivery of the rest of the head; the baby can breathe when he wishes if his nose and mouth are out of the vagina. Try to take 2–3 minutes over crowning the head.

Complications

Maternal

• Perineal tear: avoid by a properly sited episiotomy done at the right time; often an episiotomy will extend at a forceps delivery. Check for this always at the apex of the episiotomy cut.

• Damage to vagina: occasional split of vagina where caught between descending head and ischial spines.

• Retention of urine: possibly due to oedema at bladder neck. Responds to continuous drainage.

Fetal
- Bruising to head: may go on to cephalohaematoma.
- Facial palsy: facial nerve in front of ear unprotected in fetus. May be compressed by forceps blade. Usually only temporary effect.
- Intracranial haemorrhage: if blades incorrectly applied or excessive traction used.

Failed forceps
An attempt to deliver with forceps which is unsuccessful.

Reasons
1   Cervix not fully dilated.
2   Misdiagnosis of position of head. Thought to be occipitoanterior when it is occipitotransverse or occipitoposterior.
3   Unsuspected disproportion.

Treatment
Get senior help in hospital. Then:
If 1, with mother and fetus well, await full dilatation.
If 2, rotate head and deliver.
If 3, Caesarean section.

VACUUM EXTRACTOR
This instrument is used to get a purchase on the smooth fetal head, allowing traction to be applied (Fig. 6.25). The suction raises an edged dome of the soft tissues of the scalp and the pull is on the overhang of this edge.

Usage
Used widely in Europe, less in UK, least in USA.

Very useful in countries with developing health services (e.g. Africa) for it can be used by less experienced operators than forceps. With experienced doctors, combined with a division of the symphysis pubis (symphysiotomy), a baby can be delivered safely through a pelvis with too small an outlet.

Indications

First stage
1   Fetal distress after cervix is 8 cm dilated (particularly multiparous women).
2   Lack of advance after 8 cm dilated cervix (particularly multiparous women).

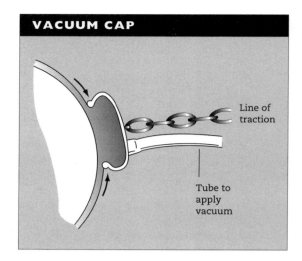

Fig. 6.25 Vacuum cap on fetal head sucks up a chignon of subcutaneous tissues to give a button on which to pull. The tractive efforts are mostly on the overhang (arrowed).

Second stage

I   Lack of advance:
   • Often with occipitoposterior or transverse position; commonly in association with an epidural.
   • Mother is too tired.

2   Compound presentations—after replacing a presenting hand.

3   High head of second twin.
   (Less use in fetal distress for forceps are swifter but, if the operator is inexperienced, the vacuum extractor is safer.)

Contra-indications
• Disproportion.
• Malpresentations (face particularly).
• Very immature infants.

Methods
This is best learned by watching and helping in the labour ward. Here essentials only are given.
• Apply largest vacuum cap that slips through cervix—60 mm if possible.
• Hold cap flat against fetal head and start to build up vacuum.
• With just enough vacuum to hold cap on head, check around the whole perimeter that maternal soft tissues have not been sucked under the cap's rim.

- Increase vacuum to 0.4 kg/cm² and again check full circumference of cap.
- Increase vacuum to 0.6 kg/cm² and again check full circumference.
- Increase vacuum to 0.8 kg/cm² and again check full circumference.
- Pull on handle, apply traction to fetal head at right angles to line of the curve of the pelvis (Fig. 6.26).
- Press cap onto head at right angles to line of traction with fingers of other hand.
- Episiotomy before head distends perineum to allow posterior pull.
- Remove cap by reducing vacuum suction.
- As well as the metal caps, there are softer rubber and Silastic caps which cause fewer fetal abrasions.

Complications

Maternal
- Cervical damage.
- Vaginal wall damage, reduced if application of cap checked so as not to suck in walls when vacuum is being established.
- Possible urinary retention later.

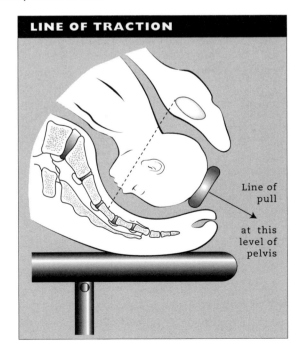

LINE OF TRACTION

Line of pull

at this level of pelvis

Fig. 6.26 Line of traction with vacuum extractor.

Fetal
- Cephalohaematoma.
- Skin abrasions.
  Both are usually minor.

CAESAREAN SECTION (CS)

Delivery of the fetus by surgical means through the abdominal wall.

Usage

Depends on availability of obstetricians and on the population served. In UK 5–15% of all deliveries.

Indications

Few are absolute, most are relative to the individual patient, the obstetrician and the obstetrical environment. Generally when the risks of vaginal delivery to the mother or baby are greater than those of abdominal delivery in any given circumstance, a CS should be done.
- Cephalopelvic disproportion.
- Fetal distress in first stage of labour or a prolapsed cord.
- Failure of labour to progress despite adequate stimulation.
- To avoid fetal hypoxia of labour: pre-eclampsia; intrauterine growth retardation.
- Antepartum bleeding: placenta praevia; abruptio placentae.
- Bad past obstetric history.
- Malpresentations: brow.
- Malpositions: transverse lie, breech.
- Death of mother in late pregnancy, a live fetus removed *post mortem*.

The only absolute ones are gross disproportion, the higher grades of placenta praevia.

In a UK population, a hospital in this decade would have the following indications for four-fifths of their operations:
- Postmaturity   15%.
- Fetal distress   15%.
- Pre-eclampsia   10%.
- Poor fetal growth   10%.
- Disorderly uterine action   10%.
- Breech, face and brow   15%.
- Previous CS   10%.

Types of approach

1 Lower segment operation: transverse approach through lower segment. In the UK over 99% of operations are lower segment because:

- Wound is extraperitoneal so less risk of intraperitoneal infection.
- Fewer postoperative complications.
- Healing of scar is better for lower segment is relatively at rest in puerperium.
- Risk of rupture less in subsequent pregnancies.

2 Classical operation: vertical approach through upper segment, performed:

- If lower segment unapproachable, e.g. fibroids; previous two or three CSs.
- If transverse lie.
- If very small baby expected (24–28 weeks), lower vertical incision (De Lee's incision).

Anaesthesia

The operation requires an anaesthetic. The alternatives are:

1 General anaesthetic.

2 Epidural block.

3 Infiltration of local anaesthetic agents.

Surgical technique

These surgical operations are best learned by watching and helping in theatre. Here only the essentials are given.

Lower segment approach

Basically for lower segment approach:

- A Pfannenstiel skin incision, low curved transverse.
- Open rectus sheath in same plane.
- Separate rectus muscles.
- Open parietal peritoneum well above bladder.
- Pick up and open loose visceral peritoneum over lower segment.
- Dislocate bladder downwards off cervix.
- Open lower segment with curved transverse approach. Watch for fetal presenting part close underneath.
- Ease out presenting part. Watch that the following shoulder does not tear the uterine wound wider.
- Divide the cord and pass baby to paediatric care (aspiration and resuscitation if required).
- Have 5 units of Syntocinon i.v. given.

- Remove placenta and membranes.
- Close uterine wound in two layers.
- Close visceral peritoneum.
- Close abdominal wall in layers.

Classical approach

- High paramedian, peri-umbilical skin incision.
- Separate rectus muscles.
- Open peritoneum to one side of mid-line.
- Check uterine rotation which is commonly to the right. Correct this manually.
- Open uterus with vertical mid-line incision through thick muscle in upper segment.
- Incise bulging membranes and extract fetal leg. Deliver rest of fetus through wound.
- Separate baby and pass to paediatric care.
- Have 5 units of Syntocinon i.v. given.
- Remove placenta and membranes.
- Close uterine wound in three layers carefully excluding dead space.
- Close abdominal wall in layers.

Complications

Haemorrhage
- Worst if angles of transverse uterine incision extend into uterine vessels.
- Always have 2 units of crossmatched blood available.

Infection
- Watch asepsis and antisepsis.
- Give prophylactic antibiotics to all women.

Abdominal distension
- Very common for a day or so.
- Await events.

Ileus
- Mild regional ileus may last 24 hours.
- Await events and avoid overloading the gut (keep on i.v. fluid for 24 hours).

Longer ileus may follow if there was a lot of handling and packing of the gut. Treat with stomach aspiration and i.v. fluids.

Pulmonary embolism
- Much higher risk after CS than after vaginal delivery.
- Avoid thrombosis by early leg exercises and mobilization.
- Avoid embolism by taking leg and pelvic signs seriously and anticoagulating early.
- Prevent thrombosis with prophylactic anticoagulation (subcutaneous heparin) in those women at higher risk:
  - (a) Aged over 35.
  - (b) Obese.
  - (c) Past history of thrombosis, particularly if oestrogen associated (e.g. oral contraception).
  - (d) Anaemia.

Prognosis

Maternal

Mortality
1 : 3000 CS with causes mostly in the above complications group.

Morbidity
Only a fifth of patients who have CS have a subsequent pregnancy. Of those that do:

1 If non-recurrent indication (e.g. fetal distress), two-thirds deliver vaginally.

2 If recurrent indication (e.g. disproportion), only one-eighth deliver vaginally.

Hence patients who have had a CS must have all subsequent pregnancies properly conducted in a hospital. Watch for dehiscence of uterine scar in late pregnancy next time. Take extra care if giving oxytocic stimulation.

Fetal

Mortality
Depends on indication; CS reduces risk, but, if done for progressive condition, it may be indicated only in the women with worse degrees of that condition and so fetal prognosis is worse, not from the operative delivery but the condition which indicated it.

Morbidity
Higher risk of retained lung fluid if delivered by CS especially before 32 weeks' gestation.

The flying squad

Every major hospital doing obstetrics in the UK used to have available obstetricians and midwives who could be taken urgently to any patient who presented with an obstetric emergency outside the hospital environment. In some teams which covered a larger area, an anaesthetist was included. The squad used to represent the patching up of a domiciliary and GP unit service. Table 6.3 shows the various reasons for an emergency call for the Flying Squad.

Much of the real service has become a resuscitation one, the woman being brought to a state suitable for transfer back to the hospital where definitive treatment takes place. Problems at delivery have almost disappeared and the squad was being called inappropriately. One-quarter of patients are given i.v. therapy but <1% had uncross-matched blood. Many of the calls related to normal women who have just delivered. The ambulance service is required to transport such women but no Flying Squad is needed, rather a community midwife or a paramedic.

The Flying Squad is a condemnation of the conditions under which domiciliary and small GP unit obstetrics were forced onto the community and is an indication of the persistence of Victorian standards in this decade's practice. Previously private transport was rare, telephones were unusual and it was hard to get to the hospital. All that is changed and now, every time obstetricians, midwives and anaesthetists have to leave the centre to look after an individual, it leaves the larger number of women at that hospital with a diminished service.

Now paramedics in the ambulance services are being trained in advanced resuscitation. They go to the home or GP unit and bring the woman safely into hospital.

REASONS FOR FLYING SQUAD CALL OUTS			
Reason for calls	1975 (%)	1989 (%)	1996
Abortions	15	20	No Flying Squad
Antepartum haemorrhage	15	5	
Delivery problems	30	3	
Normal delivery	0	70	
Postpartum haemorrhage and other third stage problems	40	2	

Table 6.2 Breakdown of calls by one Flying Squad at St George's Hospital.

A few flying squads persist in rural areas, but by 1996 most have been closed down for most of the service is a resuscitation one making better use of the skills of paramedics and not needing midwives or obstetricians.

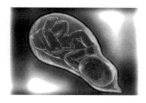

Multiple Pregnancies and Deliveries

The commonest litter size in the human species is one. Other multiples are rare (Table 7.1) and vary with racial characteristics inside the species (e.g. there is a higher incidence in West Africa than in Europe).

The differences between actual and theoretical figures are probably due to the reducing birth rate and the associated fewer births to older women and those of higher parity; both these are factors in increased multiple pregnancy rates.

Twins

TYPES (Fig. 7.1)

Monovular twins

Monovular twins are produced from one ovum fertilized by one sperm. After the two-cell division instead of going into the four-cell stage, the blastomere divides into two separate cell bodies which go on to two individuals. Thus there is common chromatin material; sex and physical characteristics will be the same, producing identical twins.

Binovular twins

Binovular twins are from two separate ova fertilized by two different sperms. These ova are shed in one menstrual cycle and most likely to be fertilized after one intercourse although they could be at separate times. The two blastomeres develop separately and have different chromatin material. They can, therefore, be of different sexes and physically have no

216

Table 7.1 Rates of multiple pregnancies per 1000 deliveries in England and Wales in 1989 compared with the biologically expected rate.

RATES OF MULTIPLE PREGNANCIES

	Actual	Theoretical
Twins	10.8	12.5 (1 : 80)
Triplets	0.24	0.16 (1 : 80^2)
Quadruplets and higher orders	0.02	0.02 (1 : 80^3)

MONOVULAR AND BINOVULAR TWINS

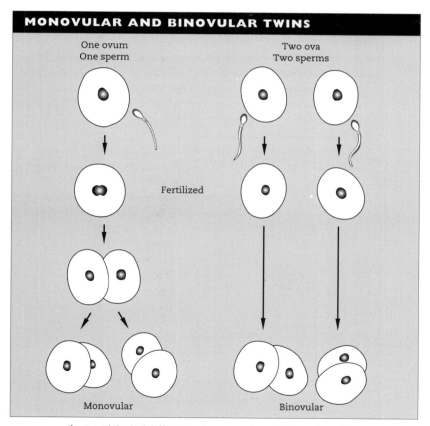

Fig. 7.1 Biological differences in monovular and binovular twins.

more in common than any other members of the same family. They are non-identical twins. Early ultrasound can help differentiation.

Incidence

Monovular twins have an incidence of 3 or 4:1000 worldwide and there is only a slight familial tendency. Binovular twins may have a family history on the maternal side. It is these that account for racial and maternal age variations. Binovular twins are more common than monovular ones (4:1). Binovular twins are commoner if:

- Maternal family history of non-identical twins.
- Over 35 years.
- After replacement of three or more fertilized ova at *in vitro* fertilization or gamete intra-Fallopian transfer procedure.

Differentiation of twins (Fig. 7.2)

1 *Sex.* If of different sexes, obviously binovular. If of one sex, may be either.

2 *Placenta.* If two separated placentae, will be binovular; if one placenta, may be monovular or binovular (Fig. 7.3). Check septum between sacs by peeling amnions from each other (Table 7.2).

3 *Blood groups.* If doubt in dichorionic types, check the ABO, Rh, Duffy, Kell and MNS.

4 *Fingerprints.* If different, binovular.

5 *DNA fingerprinting* with probes identifying about 60 dispersed sequences of variable size.

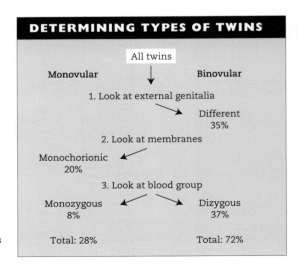

Fig. 7.2 Determining types of twins.

PLACENTAL TYPES IN TWINNING

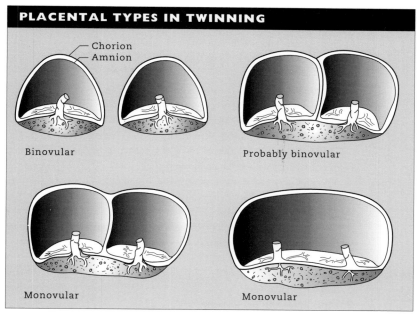

Fig. 7.3 Placental types in twinning. Often the intervening membranes can be seen in early pregnancy on ultrasound and the two types of twins differentiated.

DIFFERENTIATION OF TWINS

Septum	Placenta type	Twin type
None	Monoamniotic Monochorionic	Monovular
Amnion only	Diamniotic Monochorionic	Monovular
Amnion and chorion	Diamniotic Dichorionic	Binovular or monovular

Table 7.2 Differentiation of twins by checking placentae.

DIAGNOSIS OF TWINS

History
- Suspicion on family history especially maternal non-identical twins.
- Suspicion on past obstetric history of twins.
- Suspicion of excessive vomiting in early pregnancy.

Examination

Examination from 20 weeks onwards shows uterus bigger than expected. At first a lot of limbs are felt and later, about 30–32 weeks, more than two separate poles determined (e.g. two heads and one breech).

Investigation

Ultrasound at 6–7 weeks may show two or more sacs. The embryos can be seen in these at 7–8 weeks. The differentiation of mono from binovular can often be made by expert examination of the dividing membranes.

Commonly one of a pair of twins diagnosed early does not develop and is absorbed: the vanishing twin syndrome.

Without ultrasound, twins may not be diagnosed until delivery on rare occasions. While embarrassing to the attendants, this usually does not affect the second twin unless Syntometrine was given inadvertently at the birth of the first baby. This could jeopardize the O_2 supply to twin II and so his delivery should be speeded.

MANAGEMENT OF TWINS

Complications in pregnancy

1   Abortion is more frequent.
2   Preterm labour commoner (50% before 37 weeks).
3   Pre-eclampsia commoner ($\times$ 3).
4   Risk of anaemia increased.
   • Iron deficiency.
   • Folic acid deficiency.
5   Polyhydramnios commoner ($\times$ 10 with uniovular twins).
6   Risk of APH increased.
   • Abruptio placentae.
   • Placenta praevia.

Management in pregnancy

1   Diagnose early by bearing it in mind (one only diagnoses what one thinks about); often ultrasound will give the result before clinical suspicion.
2   Give extra iron and folic acid supplements and see that the woman takes them.
   • Check blood more often for haemoglobin levels.
3   Increased rest:
   • May prevent pre-eclampsia.
   • May prevent preterm labour.
   This may have to be in hospital if clinical signs of either of the above appear or if the patient is unable to rest at home (e.g. other children in the house).

Complications in labour

1 Prolapse of umbilical cord is more common.

2 Mechanical collision of leading parts (or locking) as they try to enter the pelvis. This is very rare.

3 Delay in delivery of twin II is associated with a higher mortality.

4 PPH is more common.

Management in labour

1 Always plan for hospital delivery.

2 Ensure twin I is longitudinal. Commonest combinations of presentations show that both twins lie longitudinally 90% of the time and the first twin is a cephalic presentation in 80% (Fig. 7.4). Noncephalic presentations are common if early preterm labour.

If twin I is transverse, do a Caesarean section.

3 Check for cord prolapse when membranes rupture (often early in labour).

4 Progress is usually uneventful. Monitor both fetal hearts and have an i.v. drip running.

5 An epidural anaesthetic is useful for it allows rapid anaesthesia for any manoeuvres that may be required for twin II in the second stage.

6 Deliver twin I appropriately. Have an anaesthetist and a paediatrician in the labour ward. Because fetus may be small, episiotomy will be required. Make sure that nobody inadvertently gives Syntometrine to the mother.

7 Clamp cord of twin I and divide. Hand baby to competent assistant or paediatrician in case resuscitation is required.

8 Immediately check the lie of twin II. If longitudinal, check presenting part. If oblique or transverse, make longitudinal.

• External version—usually easy for uterus is lax.

or

• Combined external and internal version — rupture membranes and bring a leg of the fetus down through the cervix. This produces an incomplete breech presentation but it is at least longitudinal.

9 Twin II is best delivered within 20 minutes of twin I. Usually uterus starts contracting again about 5 minutes after first delivery. If it does not do so spontaneously, use i.v. oxytocin augmentation. Very little is needed. Rupture membranes of second sac and deliver appropriately.

10 Give Syntometrine with delivery of twin II and continue oxytocin infusion for another hour.

11 Deliver placentae as soon as uterus is contracted after delivery of twin II, for retained placentae are common.

PRESENTATION OF TWINS AT DELIVERY

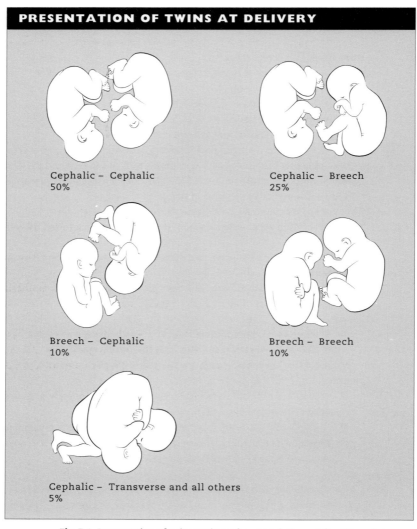

Cephalic – Cephalic
50%

Cephalic – Breech
25%

Breech – Cephalic
10%

Breech – Breech
10%

Cephalic – Transverse and all others
5%

Fig. 7.4 Presentation of twins at time of mature delivery (after 36 weeks).

Outcome

Maternal
Higher risk:
- The complications of pregnancy, e.g. pre-eclampsia.
- The complications of delivery, e.g. anaesthesia and PPH.

Fetal
• Risks of twin I are twice and twin II about three times those of single births.
Causes of death:
  (a) Immaturity.
  (b) Hypoxia.
  (c) Risks of operative delivery. } especially twin II.
• Neonatal risks are jaundice or anaemia following intrauterine shunting of blood inside the placenta leading to twin-to-twin transfusion.

Fetus papyraceus

If one twin dies late in pregnancy, his body is dehydrated and squashed by the developing other twin. This results in a *pressed flower* mini-fetus sometimes found in the membranes of an apparently singleton baby.

Triplets

Rarely due to tri-ovulation:
• Usually binovular twins with one fertilized egg dividing into two individuals.
• Usually born at an even more immature stage than twins and have double the risks.
• The complications and management are as for twins. Because of the immaturity of the fetus, delivery is commonly by Caesarean section.

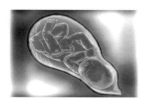

Normal Puerperium

The puerperium is the time when the mother is returning to her pre-pregnant state. The various organ systems take different times but the bulk of physical restoration has occurred by 6 weeks. During this time, one should aim at:

- Restoring maternal health and preventing illness.
- Maintaining infant health and preventing illness.
- Establishing infant feeding.
- Educating the mother about her child's and her own future health.

Physiological changes in genital tract

Uterus

Uterine bulk is reduced by involution, a rapid atrophy following withdrawal of oestrogens so that it is below the pubis by 10–12 days.

- Thrombosis of blood vessels.
- Autolysis of cellular cytoplasm of myometrium.
- Regeneration of endometrium within 2–6 weeks.
- The uterus never returns quite to nulliparous size but close to it.
- The cervix is normally stretched at delivery and the external os is altered in shape after a delivery (Fig. 8.1).

Vulva

After the stretching of labour, tissues revert to non-pregnant state with the following differences:

- Less fatty tissue in the labia.
- Hymen is wrecked leaving skin tags only (carunculae myrtiformes).
- Episiotomy or tear area leaves scar.

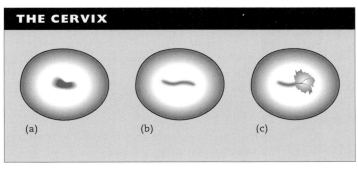

Fig. 8.1 The appearance of the cervix. (a) In the nulliparous. (b) After delivery with the usual splitting of the cervix. (c) After a more extensive laceration with an ectropion.

Management of first week

Observations

- Temperature: watch for pyrexia.
- Pulse rate: watch for transient tachycardia associated with thrombosis.
- Blood pressure: Check if pre-eclampsia occurred in pregnancy.
- Uterine size: check daily diminutions.
- Lochia: loss from vagina in the first days is the shedding of the decidua. Starts red with fresh blood but pales over 2 weeks to yellow-white. This may last for weeks.
- Urine output: normal diuresis starts within 24 hours and lasts about 3 days.
- Bowels: often constipation. Avoid too long a gap for a very hard stool is painful. Provide fibre to give bulk to stools from 1st day.
- Haemoglobin: check level about day 2 even if blood loss at delivery is recorded as minimal. Give oral iron if below 11 g/dl. Re-advise on diet.

Pain relief

Uterine contractions

- After-pains of uterine contractions are often painful and deserve analgesics.
- Warn the woman that they are coming so that she is prepared.
- Often felt more in multigravia than after first delivery.

Perineal

- After the local anaesthetic wears off, the episiotomy will hurt. Further, oedema and burning may make sitting uncomfortable. Give air ring, analgesics, local heat and, if oedematous, ice packs or hypertonic (3N) saline.
- Check sutures are not cutting in.

Sedation

See the mother gets adequate sleep. Factors against this are:

1 Excitement of new baby.
   - Sedate at night (e.g. temazepam 10–20 mg).
2 Ward noise.
   - Reduce.
3 Noise of baby.
   - Remove to nursery if mother agrees.
4 Pain.
   - Treat as above.

Bed rest

A balance must be struck between resting in bed enough to recover from the work of labour and resting so much as to allow stagnation of blood leading to deep vein thrombosis. Usually the woman's own dictates will guide.

Exercises

In association with bed rest, graduated exercises restore muscle tone to stretched areas and maintain venous flow in limbs and pelvis. Detailed regimens differ from one hospital to another. In principle they are aimed at four areas of the body:

1 Breathing exercises.
2 Legs to prevent stagnation of blood in veins.
3 Abdominal wall to restore tone of rectus muscles.
4 Pelvic floor to restore levator ani.

These are best taught by a physiotherapist who visits the patients daily and teaches them what to do after leaving hospital. Fifteen minutes twice a day is required and patients should be encouraged to continue these exercises after home going.

Diet

Adequate, nutritious and, if breast feeding, plenty of fluid.

Psychological support

Producing a baby can be a psychological stress. Women with different emotional backgrounds respond variously. Most women find a balance between the excitement and pleasure of the event on the one hand and the worry and responsibility of looking after the baby on the other. Some become apprehensive about the last factor; early reassurance and instruction in infant care will prevent a more serious problem from developing. Commonly some days after delivery there is a combination of worries about fitting the new baby into the family and discomfort from the perineum and possibly engorged breasts; this leads to a mild depression, *5th day blues*. Watch for this and prevent it by:

- Adequate explanation of what is happening to the baby.
- Night sedation.
- Pain relief.
- Getting home early.

Discharge to home

The length of postnatal stay in hospital is determined by social and manpower factors as well as by medical ones. It is reducing as the community services take up their share of looking after those who need less acute care than the hospital provides.

Many health authorities now run planned, very early discharge schemes (DOMINO: DOMestic IN and Out) where a woman comes into hospital with her community midwife, delivers and goes home a few hours later. In some instances a *birth room* is used, geographically apart but close to the labour suite; here the woman can be delivered by her midwife in less hospitalized surroundings. If an emergency arises, obstetric, anaesthetic or paediatric care is immediately available.

50% of women now leave the hospital by day 2 under planned discharge schemes evolved between the hospital and the local authority services, including community midwives and general practitioners. Those who had uncomplicated Caesarean sections go home at 3−5 days.

Advantages of earlier discharge

1   Satisfaction. By planning and letting the woman know she will return home in a short time, she is happier and more willing to be admitted to hospital for the time of maximum risk: labour.

2   Leaves more beds available for:
- *Labour* thus abolishing the idea of booking only a fixed proportion of women for hospital delivery and using high-risk factor lists to decide. The problem was always where to draw the line on a list of relative risks.
- *Antenatal complications* so that more intensive care can be directed to the fetus who is small for dates or to women with pre-eclampsia.

3   Reduces the risks of hospital infection. This is a rapidly diminishing factor in the UK but outbreaks of gastroenteritis and haemolytic streptococcal infection do still occasionally happen where babies and mothers are collected together.

Disadvantages of earlier discharge

1   Lack of rest. Household duties, particularly if there are children already in the family who soon demand the woman's attention. She is not able to do this whilst in the hospital but they rapidly impinge on her after arrival at home.

2   Poor housing conditions. If the woman is unsupported or from the lower income groups, she may be better kept in hospital for a little longer because of lack of amenities at home (e.g. easily available toilet or bath). This is a diminishing problem in the UK but a small proportion of homes (5–10%) are still considered to be unsuitable for the early reception of mothers and babies.

3   Medical problems after delivery may not be diagnosed. This is unlikely if proper community cover is given so that women who go home are visited promptly by arrangement. The medical conditions that may arise at this time are mostly well within the diagnostic powers of the local authority services. Treatment can then be decided in the home or on return to hospital as considered appropriate. In fact only a very small number of early discharged women are re-admitted for medical problems (less than 2%).

The baby

EVALUATION AT BIRTH

The most popular assessment of the newborn is the Apgar score (Table 8.1). A baby born in good condition scores nine, a less well baby two or three. This score mixes two precise observations (heart rate and respiration) with three more subjective ones. The Apgar score should not be

APGAR SCORE

Sign	Score 0	Score 1	Score 2
Heart rate	Absent	<100	>100
Respiratory effort	Absent	Irregular	Good, crying
Muscle tone	Flaccid	Some limb tone	Active
Reflex irritability	None	Cry or grimace	Vigorous cry
Colour	White	Blue	Pink

Table 8.1 Apgar score.

used as a guide to prognosis but as a description of the baby's condition at birth and response to resuscitation.

The time of onset of the first breath should also be noted.

If feasible, a sample of cord blood is taken for pH and base deficit estimation.

EXAMINATION

All newborn babies should be examined soon after delivery and a detailed examination must be done within the first 24 hours of life. The first examination should be done by the doctor or midwife in charge of the delivery:

1   To detect congenital abnormalities.

2   To detect illnesses from the antenatal or intrapartum environment, e.g. intrauterine infection, birth asphyxia, birth trauma.

3   Measure and document weight, length and head circumference.

4   Discuss baby with mother.

General observations

- Breathing pattern, check respiratory rate is <60/minutes.
- Neurological behaviour, check cry and movements.
- Check skin for pallor, cyanosis and skin blemishes.

Head

- Anterior fontanelle: check for size and tension.
- Ears: shape and position.
- Eyes: check epicanthic folds and subconjunctival haemorrhages.
- Lip and palate: check for cleft.
- Mouth: check for natal teeth and mucous cysts in mouth.

Upper limbs

- Number of digits on hands and interdigital webbing.
- Palmar creases.

Chest

- Breasts—breast enlargement is common and harmless.
- Auscultate for:
  (a) Respiratory sounds.
  (b) Heart sounds: a faint heart murmur heard during the initial examination is usually innocent. Check daily if murmur heard; investigate persistent murmurs or those associated with other signs.

Abdomen

- Umbilicus: check two arteries and one vein. Umbilical hernia.

- Palpate abdomen for liver and other masses.
- Groins:
  (a) femoral pulses.
  (b) herniae.
- Anus: check patency.

Genitalia

- Female: clitoris size (do not force labia apart).
- Male: check for hypospadias, undescended testes and hydrocele.

Back

- Myelomeningocele.
- Mid-line hairy patch, naevus or sacral pit suggests spina bifida occulta.
- Straight spine; any kyphosis or scoliosis.

Lower limbs

- Number of digits on foot.
- Talipes deformities of feet.
- Examine hips for congenital dislocation.

Measurements of body size

- Body weight.
- Occipitofrontal head circumference.
- Crown–heel length.
- Plot above on chart relating the values to gestational age.

IMMEDIATE MANAGEMENT

Temperature

Newborn babies cool rapidly and need to be kept warm.
- Dry the baby and loosely wrap in a warmed, sterile, cotton blanket.
- Draughts should be avoided.
- Room temperature after birth should be around 27°C but are often 25°C.

Infection

All babies are at a high risk of infection.
- Wipe baby clean of vernix, blood, meconium after birth.
- Bath daily after 2nd or 3rd day if baby's temperature stable.
- Watch eyes for signs of early infection.
- Watch skin flexures for moisture as; they can become excoriated.

Cord care

- Reclamp with plastic clip about 2–3 cm from umbilicus and trim to 5 cm.
- Keep dry after washing.
- Cord shrivels and mummifies.
- No dressings, for the stump dries quicker if exposed to air.
- It should separate on about the 8th–10th day.

Blood glucose

Small for dates, preterm and infants of diabetic mothers are at risk of hypoglycaemia. BM Stix should be checked regularly in these babies and any others at risk. If 2 mmol/l or less a paediatrician should be informed.

Screening tests

- The first examination in the labour ward should be repeated within 24 hours by a paediatrician or obstetrician.
- Babies of Rh-negative mothers should have blood group, haemoglobin, Coombs' test and bilirubin on umbilical cord blood at delivery.
- Guthrie test, heel prick on 6th day to detect raised level of phenylalanine indicating phenylketonuria; single spot of blood on filter paper card.
- Second spot of blood used to assay TSH. Raised level indicates hypothyroidism. If either is positive, paediatric evaluation is needed.
- Some centres screen for raised serum trypsin levels on filter paper spot. High serum trypsin is suggestive of cystic fibrosis.
- Babies a high risk for inherited disorders from a positive family history should be seen by paediatricians early and necessary treatment undertaken, e.g. cystic fibrosis, clotting disorders, inborn errors of metabolism.

FEEDING

Babies should be breast fed; in UK 60% of mothers do at first and 30% are still breast feeding at 6 weeks. Mothers should be given advice about methods of feeding in the antenatal period and breast feeding should be encouraged.

Breast

Mothers are encouraged to put the baby to the breast for a few minutes at each side. This can be done in the labour ward or certainly within 4 hours of birth.

▮ The infant will initially obtain only a small amount of colostrum when he sucks. This contains anti-infective substances. By sucking, the infant stimulates the production of more colostrum and then milk.

2   Most of the feed is obtained within the first 3–5 minutes. The time the baby is on the breast is not proportional to the amount of milk received.

3   Baby takes the nipple towards the middle of his mouth, not just between the gums.

4   The most satisfactory method of breast feeding is on demand. Babies often feed every 2–3 hours during the first few weeks and these frequent feeds stimulate lactation. A rigid regimen of feeding is not to be encouraged. Infants who are initially fed on demand usually settle down within a few weeks to a regular pattern of feeding. In general, hungry babies cry and it is difficult to overfeed a breast-fed baby.

5   If lactation is insufficient in the first few days, breast feeding should not be abandoned. Help and guidance should be given to the mother, as often breast feeding is not established until mother and baby are at home and in the 2nd week.

Factors which may help breast feeding

- Motivation: encouragement at antenatal classes.
- Proper brassiere to hold breasts correctly.
- Change nappy before feeding to have a contented baby.
- Baby awake and mother comfortable.
- Good midwife or health visitor with plenty of time to advise and check that baby fixes on nipple.
- Adequate fluid in mother's diet.

Factors which may hinder breast feeding

- Mother does not really wish to feed.
- Inverted, retracted nipples.
- Inadequate stimulation to lactation because of mixed feeding.
- Poor fixation on the nipple.
- Child with deformity of palate, tongue or lips.

Advantages of breast feeding

1   Breast milk protein, fat and solute content designed for babies.

2   Promotes infant–mother bonding.

3   Contains anti-infective agents: active white cells, macrophages, IgA, IgG and lactoferrin.

4   Eliminates risk of infection from dirty bottles.

5   Cheap.

Problems in first week

- Engorged breasts. Days 5–6 when breast feeding is uncomfortable.
- Cracked nipples.
- Excessive air swallowing during first morning feed: rapid flow of milk.

Formula or bottle milk

All cow's milk preparations in the UK are low solute milks. They have sodium and protein concentrations similar to those in human milk and most have added vitamins. Only these preparations should be used in newborn infants.

1   A normal full-term infant receives about 60 ml/kg on the 1st day of bottle feeding. This should then be increased to 150 ml/kg/day by the end of the 1st week. This is usually divided into 6 feeds/24 hours, e.g. 75 ml in each feed for a 3 kg baby.

2   Make up feeds according to instructions. If feeds are made up for 24 hours, keep in refrigerator.

3   Wash bottles and tests, then sterilize with dilute hypochloride solution.

4   When feed is due, place bottle in pan of hot water and warm milk to temperature acceptable to back of hand. However, feeding at room temperature does not cause any problems.

5   Solids should start around 4 months or earlier if the baby can take them.

Problems

1   Protein, fat and solute load not the same as human breast milk.

2   Lacks anti-infective properties of breast milk.

3   Teat hole may be too large (too much milk to cope with) or too small (too little milk).

4   Dirty bottles may lead to infections.

5   Expensive.

Postnatal visit

Conventionally the puerperium lasts 6 weeks. By then most organs have reached their resting state and infant feeding patterns have been well established.

In many centres, the woman is requested to return to the hospital outpatients for a check at this time. Response varies with the enthusiasm of the hospital staff and their handling of the woman when she was in hospital. Percentages attending range from 20 to 70% of those delivered.

Some hospitals have stopped postnatal clinics *per se*, spreading the care between:

1   Maternal medical problems—the gynaecological clinic.

2   Paediatric medical problems—the paediatric clinic.

3   Contraception—the family planning clinic.

All women have appointments for the last; 90% of women do not require to attend either of the first two but do need the third. If no post-natal clinic, they should go to their family doctor at about 6 weeks for examination to ensure normality.

At a postnatal clinic, attention should be given to maternal and neo-natal health and contraception.

Maternal health

- History of pain or bleeding *per vaginam*.
- Weight compared with pre-pregnancy level.
- Blood pressure: especially if raised in pregnancy.
- Breasts: examine for masses; if breast feeding, check good support.
- Abdominal wall tone: check if woman is doing postnatal exercises.
- Pelvic organs:

  (a) Check that the episiotomy is well healed. There should be no ten-derness at fourchette, so allowing pain-free intercourse by this time.

  (b) Position. If the uterus is retroverted, do not worry woman by remarks about its being tipped back for it may have been so always. Check that it is a mobile retroversion; if so, leave alone.

  (c) State of cervix. Commonly an ectropion is found. If no discharge, leave alone for another 8 weeks. If still present, then treat by an outpatient method, e.g. cryosurgery.

  (d) Cervical smear for cytology if not done in the last three years.

Neonatal health

- History of feeding.
- Weight. Preferably this should have been checked weekly at an infant welfare clinic and not left to 6 weeks.
- Healing of umbilicus and any circumcision.
- Development of nervous system.
- Healing of any perinatal trauma, e.g. cephalohaematomata.

Contraception

This is most important and should be discussed with every patient at post-natal clinic. Details are covered in *Lecture Notes in Gynaecology*.

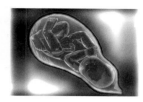

Abnormal Puerperium

Over half of maternal deaths associated with pregnancy and childbirth occur in the first few days following delivery. Although rare, this is a measure of the need for vigilance; postnatal women should be seen each day for the first 10 days by a qualified doctor or midwife.

Psychiatric problems

The baby blues

Many women feel weepy and depressed 3–5 days after delivery but this is usually short-lived (Chapter 8). The factors that prolong the baby blues are as follows:

- Postpartum pyrexia.
- Anaemia of <8 g/dl.
- Inadequate sleep.
- Delayed healing of the episiotomy or Caesarean section wound.
- Delay in establishing breast feeding.
- Decline in sympathy, congratulations and attention of friends and family as childbirth is past.

Depression

Baby blues may merge imperceptibly with serious depression. Evidence suggests that there is not a specific form of depression that is related solely to pregnancy and childbirth. The factors that aggravate depression are as follows:

- The swings in hormone changes around the time of childbirth acting on a predisposition to depression.

235

- An unconscious conflict in the responsibilities of looking after a new baby.
- Guilt.
- Anxiety.
- Fantasies.
- A background predisposition due to previous history or family history.

Treatment
- Involve a psychiatrist.
- If no psychotic delusions, can be managed as an outpatient.
- Oral antidepressants.
- Refractory cases may need definitive treatment such as electroconvulsive therapy.

Postpartum psychosis

This is a rare condition which affects 1 in 2000 women. It is potentially life-threatening to both the mother and the baby.

Symptoms
- Rejection of the baby.
- Delusion.
- Confusion.

Management
1 Admit the mother and baby to a special ward in the psychiatric unit.
2 Ensure 24 hours supervision.
3 Give appropriate psychotherapy drugs.

Postpartum psychosis is recurrent (about 20%) but chances are decreased by a 2-year or more gap between pregnancies.

Postpartum pyrexia

A temperature of over 38°C on over two occasions more than 4 hours apart. The causes are:
1 Infections of the genital tract.
2 Urinary tract infection.
3 Breast infections.
4 Thromboembolic episodes.

GENITAL TRACT INFECTION

An ascending infection which largely involves the placental bed. Unlike pelvic inflammatory disease (PID) it spreads directly through the uterus to the parametrium tissues (Fig. 9.1).

The organisms that are usually responsible for the infection are:

- *E. coli.*
- *Streptococcus faecalis.*
- *Staphylococcus.*
- Anaerobes.
- Group B haemolytic *Streptococcus.*

Diagnosis

History
- Puerperal pyrexia.
- Offensive discharge.

ROUTES OF INFECTION

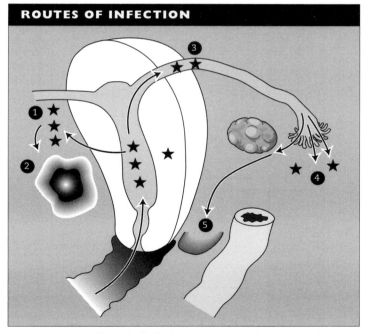

Figure 9.1 Routes of spread of infection. 1, Direct spread to parametrium—typical of postpartum endometritis and 2, the formation of pelvic abscess; 3, intracavity spread causing salpingitis or 4, sub-ovarian abscess and 5, finally spread to pouch of Douglas is more characteristic of PID in those not recently pregnant.

- Low abdominal pain.
- Passage of clots and a return of red lochia.
- Systemic symptoms associated with the temperature.

Examination
- Raised temperature and pulse.
- Bulky uterus.
- Tender uterus.
- Offensive lochia (often bleeding with clots).
- An open internal cervical os.

Investigations
- Hb—may be reduced.
- White cell count—shows a neutrophilia.
- High vaginal swab—may grow the organisms.

Management
1   Admit to hospital.
2   Evacuation of retained products of conception under antibiotic cover.
    Broad-spectrum antibiotics should be used to cover the bacteraemia
and subsequently for 5 days.

Complications

Acute (see Fig. 9.1)
- Parametritis.
- Broad ligament abscess.
- Salpingitis.
- Peritonitis.
- Septic thromboembolism.

Longer-term
- Infertility.
- Menstrual irregularities and pelvic pain.

URINARY TRACT
These are common in the puerperium because:
1   Bladder stasis due to temporary nerve damage (neuropraxia).
2   Oedema of the bladder base.
3   Diminished bladder sensation.
4   Catheterization in labour.
    The commonest organisms are *E. coli* and *Proteus*.

Diagnosis

History
- Dysuria.
- Frequency of micturition.
- Loin pain of pyelonephritis supercedes.
- Systemic symptoms such as pyrexia and tachycardia.
- May be asymptomatic and recognized on routine MSU which should be performed on all patients who have been catheterized in labour.

Examination
- Raised temperature.
- Tender suprapubically or in the renal angle.
- May be no signs.

Investigations
- MSU.
- White cell count.

Management
- Bed rest.
- High fluid, light solid diet.
- Broad-spectrum antibiotics until the results of culture and sensitivity are known, then be specific.

Complications
- Pyelonephritis.
- Exacerbation of the baby blues.

BREAST INFECTION

This usually enters through a break in the skin (cracked nipple). It is usually confined to one quadrant of the breast. Most commonly it is due to *Staphylococcus aureus*.

Diagnosis

History
Painful area of one breast.

Examination
- Raised temperature.
- Erythematous segment of the breast.
- If an abscess, brawny swelling or even fluctuation.

Investigation

Send some expressed breast milk from the affected side for bacteriological examination.

Management

Without abscess

1 Supportive brassiere.

2 Continue breast feeding or empty the breast by means of a breast pump.

3 Give an antistaphylococcal antibiotic such as flucloxacillin.

With abscess

1 Incise under a general anaesthetic.
- Circumareola incision.
- Break down lochia and leave a drain through dependent part.

2 Adequate supportive brassiere.

3 Appropriate antibiotics.

THROMBOEMBOLISM

The postpartum period is the commonest time in pregnancy for a thromboembolism as the puerperium fulfils all the criteria of Virchow's triad:

1 *Increased coagulation.* The increase in clotting factors from pregnancy remains although plasma volume returns to normal within a few hours of delivery.

2 *Stasis.* Many women are immobilized during labour or the immediate puerperium.

3 *Damage to venous endothelium.*
- Uterine veins—when placenta separates.
- Deep leg veins—when weight of legs continues to compress veins if woman is immobilized in bed.

Diagnosis

History
- Calf pain.
- Unilateral leg oedema.

Examination
- A low-grade postpartum pyrexia.
- An unexplained maternal tachycardia.

- Tenderness over the deep veins of the calf.
- A positive Holman's sign (calf tenderness on foot dorsiflexion).

Investigations

Doppler ultrasound
- Simple continuous wave Doppler ultrasound will fail to show flow in the femoral vein.
- Colour flow Doppler may actually demonstrate the clot within the veins.

Venography
- This is the definitive test and should be performed whenever the diagnosis is suspected clinically using image intensifiers and low-viscosity contrast medium.
- Radioisotope scanning. This is contra-indicated antenatally but may be used in the puerperium. Microaggregates of radiotagged albumen or microspheres labelled with radio technetium accumulate behind the clot and may be demonstrated with a gamma counter system.

Management

Prevention
1   Early mobilization—all recently delivered women are encouraged to be up and about as soon as they wish.
2   High-dose oestrogens no longer given to suppress breast milk.
3   Prophylaxis is usually given to women who have had a previous history of thromboembolism.
- Compression stockings worn during labour or Caesarean section.
- Subcutaneous heparin.
- Dextran i.v.

Treatment
1   Anticoagulate immediately with full dose i.v. heparin given by means of a continuous infusion pump. This prevents further extension of the venous thrombosis with a possible risk of pulmonary embolism.
2   Long-term anticoagulation with warfarin for 12 weeks. The period of 10 days for i.v. heparin is chosen for the following reasons:
- Warfarin therapy in the puerperium is difficult to control.
- There is evidence that i.v heparin allows earlier recanalization of the clotted veins.

Pulmonary embolism

The most dangerous of the common resting places of a clot embolus from the soleal or pelvic veins is in the pulmonary circulation.

I *Mild cases* follow microemboli. Dyspnoea and slight, poorly defined pleural pain. The condition resolves in a few days with no specific treatment.

2 *Severe cases* arise from clot from the:
- Soleal veins—clot extends to populiteal vein and breaks off (30%).
- Uterine and ovarian veins — a thrombophlebitis with a friable clot following mid pelvic sepsis (20%).

In 50%, no clinical signs exist before the pulmonary embolism.

Diagnosis

History
Pre-existing deep vein thrombosis (in half the cases only).
At first:
- Acute dyspnoea.
- Faintness.

Later:
- Chest pain.
- Haemoptysis.

Examination
At first:
- No physical signs beyond dyspnoea.

Later:
- May be cyanosis.
- Local signs of pulmonary underperfusion.
- Right heart failure.

Later still:
- Pleural signs.
- Collapse of a pulmonary lobe.

Investigations
Often no positive tests early. Next day:
I X-ray:
- Raised diaphragm on affected side.
- Consolidation and infiltration of lung(s).

2 ECG—rhythm disturbance.
- Lead I—S wave inversion.

- Lead III—T wave inversion and deep Q wave.
- Leads V1, 2, 3, 4—T wave inversion.
- Excludes cardiac infarction.

3 Lung scan with radioactive albumin to show ischaemic areas.
4 Pulmonary angiography to show clot.
5 Left and right heart catheterization to show reversal of pressures.

The last three are used in specialist thoracic units.

Management

Two-thirds of those dying do so within 2 hours, so act quickly on suspicion, not awaiting the sophisticated tests even if they are very easily available.

Resuscitation if required

1 External cardiac massage.
2 Positive pressure O_2 by intubation if necessary.
3 Heparin 40 000 units i.v. a day.
4 Emergency embolectomy—only in hospitals with their own thoracic units with bypass facilities.

Definitive treatment

If resuscitation is successful, give:

1 Anticoagulants (more i.v. heparin):
  - 25 000 units immediately.
  - 25 000 units 6-hourly for 24 hours.

  This is to prevent further emboli.

  Then warfarin oral therapy controlled by prothrombin time.

2 Thrombolytics (streptokinase). Actively accelerate lysis of existing clot:
  - 500 000 units immediately.
  - 100 000 units hourly for 72 hours.

3 Embolectomy (mortality rate 25%). Useful if:
  - Thoracic unit in the same hospital.
  - No response to streptokinase.
  - Too ill for streptokinase.
  - Contra-indication to streptokinase, e.g. recent surgery, peptic ulcer or hypertension.

Both high-dose heparin and streptokinase have high risk of bleeding. Not indicated unless embolus is thought to be life-threatening. If started, reduce to conservative dosage in 2–3 days and continue for 4–6 weeks.

Secondary postpartum haemorrhage

Any considerable fresh bleeding occurring in the puerperium after 24 hours. This is dealt with in Chapter 6.

Previous diseases continuing into the puerperium

PRE-ECLAMPSIA AND ECLAMPSIA

When these conditions occur before delivery, their ultimate treatment is delivery of the baby. Usually the woman gets better rapidly after the placenta is delivered and the normal diuresis starts to remove the water/salt overload. A few women stay as bad or worsen in the first few days of the puerperium. Management is the same as in pregnancy. Postpartum eclampsia has a high mortality rate.

DIABETES

Delivery may be operative and for a day immediately after the women may be on i.v. therapy. Remember that insulin requirements drop very sharply in the puerperium so that many diabetics are at their pre-pregnant level by 2 days into the puerperium. Infection of any wounds is more likely and breast feeding may be an irregular drain of carbohydrates, making insulin balance more difficult.

HEART DISEASE

The first 24 hours of the puerperium are dangerous, for the post-delivery shunting of blood from the uterine vessels may lead to pulmonary oedema and subsequent right-sided cardiac failure. After that the risk is reduced.

Puerperal infection could release bacteria that might colonize on any damaged endothelium in the heart (acute bacterial endocarditis). This is more likely to follow a congenital heart disease than rheumatic conditions but antibiotic cover is often provided for either in the puerperium.

OVARIAN TUMOURS

These are more likely to undergo torsion in the puerperium because of the lax abdominal wall and the diminishing uterus. Surgery is recommended for any ovarian masses above 10 cm diameter.

Maternal mortality

Definition
Death of a woman associated with pregnancy, or with childbirth within 42 days of that event.

Causes
Maternal death is often straightforward to attribute (e.g. a massive PPH) but, as well as those occurring as a direct result of obstetrical complications or their treatment in pregnancy, there are those indirectly associated with pregnancy. They are previous existing diseases which deteriorate in pregnancy. There is a third group (e.g. women killed in motor car accidents or who committed suicide) which are fortuitous deaths.

When looking at international comparative figures, the groups which are included under the definition must be remembered. Some countries exclude deaths following abortion from maternal mortality results.

Progress
Internationally, maternal deaths have fallen for the last 30 years. In the UK they are now at the level of 9.8:100 000 births. This could be expressed as 0.0098% but, since this is difficult to comprehend, it is better expressed per 100 000 births (Fig. 9.2). It may be that in the next few years the denominator will move up to a million. Then the rate will be 9.8:1 000 000 births. Figure 9.3 shows the decline of maternal deaths caused by puerperal sepsis.

The reduction may be due to:
1   Improved health of the population.
    • A more robust mother with less disease.
2   Changes in reproductive patterns:
    • Smaller families, therefore lower parity.
    • Fewer very young mothers.
    • Fewer older mothers.
3   Better education of the mothers.
    • An increased willingness to accept medical care.
4   Advances in medical knowledge.
    • Better understanding and application of physiology and pharmacology in pregnancy and delivery.
5   Improved antenatal and delivery services.
    • More better-trained doctors and midwives grouped in delivery centres.

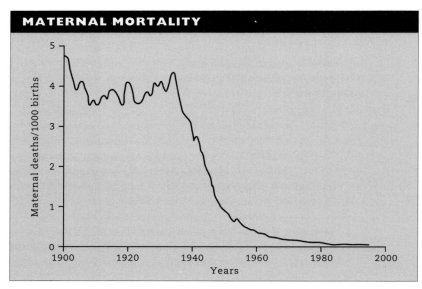

Fig. 9.2 Maternal mortality in England and Wales, 1900–1994.

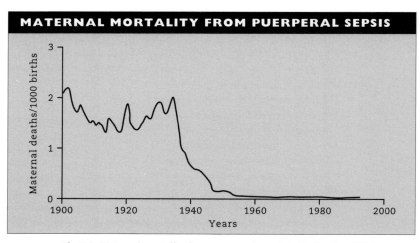

Fig. 9.3 Maternal mortality from puerperal sepsis in England and Wales, 1900–1993.

MAJOR CAUSES OF MATERNAL MORTALITY

Pre-eclampsia and eclampsia

Eclampsia is getting rarer. When it comes earlier in pregnancy (before 28 weeks) it has a worse effect. Death is from intracranial haemorrhage or renal failure.

To reduce deaths:

- Check blood pressure frequently in pregnancy.
- Insist on rest for those with early signs of pre-eclampsia.

This may be at home for lesser degrees rather than in hospital.

Pulmonary embolism

1 A third are antenatal and two-thirds after delivery. A third of the latter follow Caesarean section.

2 High-risk patients:

- Over 35 years.
- Obese.
- Operative delivery.
- Previous thrombosis.

3 Half the deaths are with little warning of previous thrombotic episodes.

To reduce deaths:

- Prophylactic anticoagulation of high-risk patients.
- Prompt effective treatment on suspicion.

Abortion

1 Usually after procured and illegal interferences.

2 Patients die from haemorrhage, sepsis or renal failure.

To reduce deaths:

- Wider use of legal therapeutic abortion.
- Better contraception.

Haemorrhage

Abruptio placentae

Severe hypovolaemia leads to shock and later renal shutdown.

To reduce deaths:

- Central venous pressure monitoring.
- Adequate and quick blood replacement.

Placenta praevia

Repeated and increasing haemorrhage in last trimester of pregnancy. The severe degrees must be treated by Caesarean section, which may be a technically difficult operation.

   To reduce deaths:
- Pay more attention to warning bleeds in pregnancy.
- Have consultant in theatre for CS.

Postpartum haemorrhage

Usually from an atonic uterus but can follow cervical trauma.

   To reduce deaths:
- Give oxytocic drug routinely at delivery.
- Deliver patients in hospital where blood is available.
- Act promptly using a planned protocol.

Ectopic pregnancy

With reductions of deaths from other forms of haemorrhage this is becoming relatively more important.

   To reduce deaths:
- Admit patients with suspicious symptoms.
- Act promptly on patients with actual symptoms.
- Be prepared to laparoscope on suspicion and do not rely on ultrasound findings alone.

Anaesthesia

Deaths associated with general anaesthesia are reducing greatly in the UK. Inhalation of acid stomach contents in labour under general anaesthetic leads to Mendelson's syndrome.

   To reduce deaths:
- Wider use of regional anaesthetics (e.g. epidural).
- If general anaesthetic essential, a senior anaesthetist gives it and intubates with a cuffed tube.

Other causes

All the other causes produce few deaths. Infection, once the killer of 1 : 10 women in childbirth, is much reduced (although still causing some deaths each year, mostly after Caesarean section in labour with long ruptured membranes). Heart disease as a cause is diminishing, as rheumatic fever is better avoided or diagnosied and treated in childhood.

SUBSTANDARD CARE

In the UK every maternal death is reported by the District Medical Officers to a central committee which publishes its confidential finds at 3-yearly intervals. This is not a judicial enquiry and no blame is apportioned to any individual. It is a medical assay where the profession looks closely at its own work and tries to learn from mistakes. The committee tries to assess in each case if an avoidable factor was present: if there was 'some departure from the acceptable standards of satisfactory care'.

In a recent report, 45% of the deaths directly due to pregnancy and delivery were considered to have been avoidable by this definition. It was the patient who made the largest single contribution to this in the antenatal period by either not coming for care or else ignoring advice given. In labour, the hospital obstetricians and anaesthetists had the highest incidence of substandard care incidents. This was mostly from not paying sufficient heed to warning signs and not having senior enough doctors in the delivery suite. Shortage of staff and facilities are beginning to be reported in this category. Substandard care from general practitioners and midwives in these cases was rare.

The most important ways of reducing maternal deaths are:
1   Better patient education.
2   Better consultant involvement in delivery unit.
3   Better antenatal care.

Perinatal mortality

The perinatal mortality rate (PMR) is the total of stillbirths and 1st-week neonatal deaths occurring in every 1000 total births. In 1994 it was 7.8/1000 total births in England and Wales.

Factors influencing PMR
1   The health of mothers.
2   The mother's:
    • Place of residence.
    • Past nutrition and diseases.
    • Education.
    • Social class.
3   The age and parity of the mother.
4   An efficient health service.
5   The definition of stillbirth and neonatal death. In the UK this was changed in 1991 to deaths after 24 completed weeks of gestation from a previous 28 weeks' limit. Hence, a small apparent increase for a short time appears.

Figure 11.4 shows the progressive reduction of PMR in 50 years.

Causes of perinatal mortality
Precise causes of perinatal death are often confused by a lack of autopsy

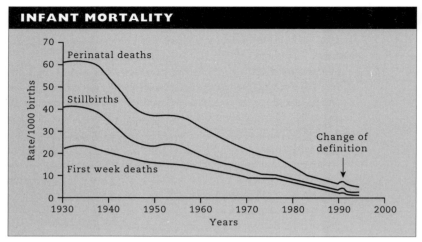

Fig. 9.4 Perinatal mortality, stillbirths and 1st-week neonatal deaths in England and Wales from 1930.

information and an insistence on a single or primary cause of death on the certificate.

Classification of causes of perinatal death
1   Macerated stillbirths without malformation.
2   Congenital malformation in either stillbirths or neonatal deaths.
3   Intrapartum perinatal deaths secondary to asphyxia or trauma or both.
4   Neonatal deaths as a result of immaturity.
5   Other specific causes, e.g. Rh haemolytic disease.

SGA
Two-thirds of neonatal deaths are associated with SGA. A high incidence of hyaline membrane disease and intraventricular haemorrhage is found.

Congenital malformations
A tenth of stillbirths and a third of neonatal deaths have a congenital anomaly. Malformations of the CNS and cardiovascular systems are the most common.

Asphyxia
There is post-mortem evidence of asphyxia in a third of stillbirths and a tenth of neonatal deaths. This is due to:

Before labour
1   Abruptio placentae.
2   Placental failure:
      • Pre-eclampsia.
      • Hypertension.
      • Post-maturity.
      • Diabetes.

In labour
1   Prolonged labour.
2   Cord prolapse.

At delivery
• Impacted shoulders.
• Delayed onset of respiration.

Birth injury
Less than a tenth of neonatal deaths.

Associated with
1   Too fast a delivery:
      • Precipitate delivery with immature fetus.
      • Breech presentation with insufficient time for moulding of head.
2   Too difficult a delivery:
      • Disproportion.
      • Badly performed operative delivery, particularly forceps.

Infection
1   Intrauterine.
2   Neonatal.

Management of perinatal death

When pregnancy ends with the loss of a fetus or a neonate, particular care and support are needed for the couple involved. This is a difficult situation not only for the parents but also for relatives, and the medical and nursing staff. Grief reactions commonly involve the following phases:
1   Initial denial of what has occurred.
2   Attempt to apportion blame to themselves.
3   Attempt to apportion blame to the doctors and midwives.
4   Eventual acceptance of their loss which may take several months.

Medical problems associated with intrauterine death
- Disseminated intravascular coagulopathy (DIC) if fetus retained for some weeks.
- Intrauterine infection.
- Difficult induction of labour.
- Psychological and possibly psychiatric sequelae.

Management of labour

1   Confirm the diagnosis of intrauterine death by means of real-time ultrasound.

2   Give the parents time to come to terms with their loss.

3   Plan induction of labour at a time that is suitable for the parents but ensuring that they have a midwife to look after them throughout the period of induction.

4   Arrange facilities for the partner to stay throughout the procedure.

Investigations

1   Hb and save serum.

2   Kleihauer test.

3   Clotting studies.

Management

1   Induce labour with prostaglandin pressaries given every 3 hours.

2   Do not rupture the membranes until the worman is in labour and the cervix is more than 4 cm dilated.

3   Keep an accurate fluid balance chart.

4   Give liberal analgesia. If the woman wishes an epidural, ensure her blood clotting values are normal.

5   Discuss whether the couple wish to see the baby after delivery. Parents should be encouraged but not pressed to view their babies.
- The babies should be photographed, clothed and looking as natural as possible. These photographs should be filed in case parents wish to see them much later—sometimes they ask a year or so later.

Postnatal care

The woman should be looked after by midwifery staff known to her in the antenatal period. The length of hospital stay is not determined by medical events but more by what the couple wish. She may go home as soon as she wishes but should not have the feeling of being sent away. Her general practitioner and community midwife must be informed of the loss of her baby by telephone.

1   Arrange for her to be seen by a specialist midwife who is skilled in counselling patients who have lost their babies.

2   Ask if she wishes her baby to be baptized and buried; if so, arrange the procedure with the hospital chaplain.

3   Consent for post-mortem should be obtained from the parents. The reason for post-mortem should be carefully explained but, if post-mortem is refused, the following procedures should be undertaken:

(a) Heart blood should be sent for karyotyping and viral studies.

(b) Two polaroid photographs of the baby should be taken. One should ba a general photograph and the other should be a close-up of the baby's face.

(c) X-ray the baby.

4   The consultant should interview the parents before discharge from hospital and explain as far as possible the circumstances surrounding the death.

5   The couple are met 4–6 weeks later with all the evidence to hand.

6   The couple should be put in touch with a society, e.g. Stillbirth, Abortion and Neonatal Death Society (SANDS), or people who have experienced a similar problem.

7   Lactation should be suppressed by means of a firm supporting brassiere. If this is insufficient, bromocriptine may be used.

8   Women who have had a hysterectomy or have one surviving twin may need professional psychotherapeutic help.

Index

Page references in *italics* refer to Figures; those in **bold** refer to Tables; boxes are indicated by the page number followed by (box)